STILL LOOKING FOR A SOLUTION
TO LOSING WEIGHT?
You might be sugar sensitive.

- Do you hate how you look?
- Are you overly sensitive to criticism or easily hurt?
- Have you tried every diet in the world, even taken medication for weight loss?
- Do you crave sugary and "white" foods, like breads and other carbohydrates?
- Do you start things and never finish them?
- Do you feel everything will be okay once you are thin?
- Do you feel foggy-headed or depressed, or do you take antidepressants?
- Do you eat compulsively or spend large amounts of energy trying not to?
- Does your struggle with your weight consume your days?

If you answered "yes" to two or more of these questions, you may be sugar sensitive. And this will be *your last diet!* *Heal those cravings and lose the weight—permanently.*

By Kathleen DesMaisons, Ph.D.

Potatoes Not Prozac

The Sugar Addict's Total Recovery Program

Your Last Diet!:
The Sugar Addict's Weight-Loss Plan

Your Body Speaks

YOUR *Last* DIET!

The Sugar Addict's Weight-Loss Plan

Kathleen DesMaisons, Ph.D.

BALLANTINE BOOKS

NEW YORK

A Ballantine Book
Published by The Ballantine Publishing Group

www.ballantinebooks.com

Library of Congress Catalog Control Number: 2002092905

ISBN 0-345-44135-4

Cover design by Michael Stromberg

Manufactured in the United States of America

First Hardcover Edition: December 2001
First Trade Paperback Edition: December 2002

10   9   8   7   6   5   4   3   2   1

Mother, your relentless demand to speak the truth and
bring healing has sustained me and nourished me.
Thanks for reminding me always
why I do this work.

Contents

Acknowledgments

This book started as an ebook published on the Web. I had written about sugar sensitivity and sugar addiction in my first two books and had then set up a website at www.radiantrecovery.com to support the development of a worldwide healing community.

Thousands of people did the recovery programs diligently. And they came back and said, "Now we are balanced and clear. But we are still fat. We need a diet book."

Your Last Diet! became a living process, and the feedback and experience of those doing it shaped its development. This book is a point-in-time snapshot of a powerful, healing, and extraordinary process. My deepest thanks go to the men and women who are members of the *Your Last Diet!* community. Your voices have guided and informed me every step of the way.

I am deeply indebted to the members of the radcounsel, volunteers who have committed to the growth and smooth sailing of the website. They, along with a group of people serving as liaisons to our many listservs and answering the thousands of letters I receive, have helped to create the miracle you will read. Fourteen women have made it possible for me to manage a website that has thousands of visitors daily and has had more than 10 million hits to it. They are Simone Baroke, Michelle Benson, Martha Carnahan, Cheryl Cunningham, Michele LoPresti, Suzanne Miller, Kitty Morel, Gretel O'Brien, Jan Potter, Allison Schacht, Jeanne Vaillaincourt, Laurie Warner, Marie Yacuzzo, and Gail Zuskin.

I continue to be deeply grateful to my agent, Ned Leavitt, who made the connection to Ballantine. Leslie Meredith, my editor par excellence, helped to craft this manuscript into something I am truly proud of. It has gone way beyond the original idea of a good, effective diet book and beome a message of real hope for those who have tried everything.

Introduction

You have read all of the diet books as soon as they were published, and you have tried a hundred diets, but you still struggle to lose weight. It seems like every month there's a new explanation for your weight gain: carbohydrate addiction, emotional eating, serotonin solutions, eating right for your blood type, balancing ratios, seeking the Zone, sugar-busting, counting calories, counting fat grams, even eating a potato before bed! You want to lose weight permanently, but what you have been doing isn't working. You are still overweight, you are in pain, and you don't know what to do. You are ready for a solution that works.

Your Last Diet! is unlike any other book you have read. It outlines how your body chemistry is different—why you feel the way you do, why you have a problem with saying no, why you seem to gain weight even though you eat less, why your moods fluctuate so much. *Your Last Diet!* teaches you *why* you are fat and what to do about it. You will learn about sugar sensitivity and understand why you crave sugar and fat so much. You will learn about your unique brain and body chemistry—why your blood sugar levels fluctuate, how the chemicals serotonin and beta-endorphin have different effects in your brain, how insulin resistance and fatty acid mobilization hold your weight on you. It is *not* your fault that you continue to struggle with your weight. You are not weak-willed and undisciplined. The problem is a function of your unique biochemistry, *not* a defect in your character. **The problem is biochemical, and you can heal.**

Your Last Diet! is the last diet you will ever have to do. It changes everything. You will shift from an obsession with the scale into an interactive, dynamic relationship with your body. You will lose weight and create the body that matches the ideal image you have of yourself. As Anne Marie wrote after she had been doing the program for six months:

> *I'm tellin' ya, it's a miracle! Plain and simple and outstanding! . . . You cannot believe the freedom that comes when you are following the program. . . . After years of living in the hell of being overweight, it just seemed impossible to get out. Yet on this program, I understand now why after years of suffering, I'm waking up feeling good, motivated, silly, happy! I'm beginning to be the person I really am.*

Your Last Diet! goes to the heart of why you are fat. Its simplicity and effectiveness seem miraculous, but *Your Last Diet!* is not glamorous—it does not promise a quick loss of thirty pounds in thirty days. It goes to the *cause* of your weight gain—the chemical imbalance of your brain and your body—and gives you the tools you need to restore the balance. The science in *Your Last Diet!* lets you finally make sense of your own body and do something to fix it. You will heal your sugar-sensitive body chemistry and *then* lose weight. The weight will come off slowly and will stay off.

Even more important, the shame you have about your weight and your body image will heal. The feelings of hopelessness and inadequacy will disappear. Your self-esteem will rise dramatically, and you will feel empowered to stick with your food plan and keep going. You will feel great because everything will have changed. You will have the body you want, and know this is the last diet you will ever do.

Your Last Diet!

1

The Problem of Sugar Sensitivity and Weight

You are fat, and diets haven't worked for you. You want to lose weight and not gain it back. You have been motivated to lose weight your entire life. You have tried every diet on earth, from the cottage cheese and grapefruit diet to the cabbage diet. It is all you think about. How can you try so hard and still not have the results you deserve? You know people who decide to diet, lose weight, and that is the end of it. Why is it so different for you?

You may be sugar sensitive. This physical and chemical condition changes everything. Take this test for sugar sensitivity. If you answer yes to three or more questions, you are reading the right book. If none of these apply to you, stop here. This is not the solution for you.

❑ You have tried every diet in the world but cannot sustain your commitment.
❑ You try again and again to cut down or control your use of sweet foods.

❑ You feel everything will be okay once you are thin.
❑ You are easily hurt.
❑ You are overly sensitive to criticism.
❑ You need a regular dose of sugar or you get irritable and cranky.
❑ You love office supply stores.
❑ You know what a "sugar hangover" is.
❑ You start things and do not finish them.
❑ You sometimes go blocks out of your way to get something sweet.
❑ You have twenty projects going on simultaneously.
❑ You have several sets of clothes—one fat set and one hopeful set.
❑ You hate how you look.
❑ You pretend that big is beautiful, but you know this is hooey.
❑ You are impulsive.
❑ You like to skip breakfast because it gives you a "starvation high," but you're famished by eleven o'clock and exhausted after lunch.
❑ Your mother bought your clothes in husky sizes.
❑ You get overwhelmed easily.
❑ You wait for new magazines to find one more diet that will work.
❑ You have taken medication for weight loss.
❑ You have taken antidepressants.
❑ Your friends tell you that you look fine, but you feel fat and ugly.

If you have answered yes to three or more of these questions, you are in the right place. You will get answers that will help you understand why you are fat, why you feel the way you do, and what you can do about it. (If you are wondering about the office supply store question, that question comes from a serendipitous discovery made in our online community at www.radiantrecovery.com. We got into an exchange about office supply stores and discovered that we all loved them. It was a little creepy at first, since we had all felt this was a personal idiosyncrasy and not a shared characteristic. But over time, we have come to love this little indicator as a secret code.)

Characteristics of Sugar Sensitives

I have spent the past ten years developing and writing about the theory of sugar sensitivity—that some people are born with a different biochemistry that makes them more vulnerable to the addictive properties of sugar and alcohol. Sugar-sensitive people have lower levels of the brain chemicals that create the simple state of feeling good. They are likely to be impulsive, have a hard time saying no, struggle with mood swings, are more vulnerable to depression, and struggle with sugar addiction. Their self-esteem fluctuates with what they eat. Sugar-sensitive people also tend to be smart, intuitive, creative, funny, compassionate, and tenacious.

The contradiction between the difficult and wonderful parts of being sugar sensitive creates a significant dilemma. You may ask yourself, "How can I be such a nice person and do such dumb things?" Even more relevant to this discussion, you may ask yourself, "How can I know so much and still be fat?"

The pain of the dissonance between all that you know and what you are actually able to do in your life is horrible. You feel guilty, hopeless, and overwhelmed. So the struggle for control over your weight and your life gets bigger, and you feel more out of control as time goes on. Food—particularly sweet food, high-fat food, and white things (refined flour products)—seems to be the only thing that comforts you and quiets the emotional pain you are in. Intellectually, you may know that the thing that seems to comfort you is actually killing you.

But you can't find a way out of compulsive eating. And you feel a profound shame about your weight that you rarely talk about. The shame is always there, sort of like an aftertaste, right under the surface. It doesn't matter what you say on the outside. It doesn't matter how much work you have done to accept yourself just the way you are. How much you weigh isn't the issue so much as this shame, this pain of your inability to control it. It follows you everywhere. You can be walking down the sidewalk and see a reflection of yourself in a plate-glass window, and all your molecules cringe. You look away in pain, then glance back again at your reflected image. "How can I *look* this way?" comes the voice inside. All your pain floods through you. The anguish of feeling fat, ugly, and out of control washes over you.

I have been in that place. When I decided to write a weight loss book, I knew I would be writing from my heart and my healing as well as my clinical experience. I know this shame and hopelessness from a deeply personal level. Before I did this program I weighed close to 265, but in my first book I said I weighed 240. Lying about your weight is part of the shame. I no longer feel it. I want you to have the healing that I have created. I want you not only to understand the science that will free you from blame but to have the joy and gratitude that come from healing your sugar-sensitive body.

I've been on *Your Last Diet!* for five and a half months, and I have so much to thank you for. On one level, you have taught me how to listen to my body, how to do what's good for it in a way that I can do comfortably. I have hope. I started from a hopeless, helpless, and scared place. Now I feel effective. Either I know what to do or I know how to find out what to do, and I realize that my progress happens in slow, steady, doable steps.

I trust my body now. This is so big for me. I had lost trust in my body. Now I know how to listen to it and take care of it, and through that connection I have built trust.

My negative, desperate thinking regarding food has changed. I have positive and hopeful thoughts now. I no longer have irresistible urges to eat things that are not good for me. In fact, I don't even really care about them.

And most important to me, I have moved out of fear into a place of compassion and confidence as my skills continue to grow in your program. I feel like I finally have the rest of the tools to take good care of myself—mind, body, and spirit.

Stephanie

If this is the first time you have heard about sugar sensitivity and you want to heal this condition and lose weight, *Your Last Diet!* is for you. The solution in *Your Last Diet!* changed my life and the lives of more than four thousand people who are connected through our community at www.radiantrecovery.com. It has helped people who are fat or just in need of trimming.

My first book, *Potatoes Not Prozac,* gives an in-depth discussion of the theory of sugar sensitivity and was the first to lay out the seven steps. It connects food and mood in a unique way. My second book, *The Sugar Addict's Total Recovery Program,* explains the relationship of sugar sensitivity to sugar addiction and provides a detailed road map for healing your body on a day-to-day basis.

Your Last Diet! takes the information one step further into weight loss. While some sugar sensitives have lost weight doing the food plans of my first two books, some did not. *Your Last Diet!* will help this latter group. Some others may have lost weight and then reached a plateau and are not losing any more. *Your Last Diet!* will also help them.

Key Issues for You

Being sugar sensitive and overweight brings a history with many variables. It is too shortsighted to say that you simply need to lose weight and be done with it. I am interested in healing your body and then helping you get to your ideal weight. Let's take a look at what may be going on for you.

- You are overweight or fat and cannot lose weight.
- You are fat and cannot maintain your weight loss.
- You have a long history of dieting.
- You love sugar, carbohydrates, and fats.
- You are sugar sensitive.
- You are insulin resistant.
- You have a body with unique biochemical responses.

Before we look at the biochemistry of why you are overweight, let's talk some about sugar sensitivity and examine what it is and how it affects your moods and your behavior. "Sugar sensitivity" is a term I coined to describe a three-part syndrome that I believe is inherited and includes these three components:

- Volatile blood sugar
- Low levels of the brain chemical serotonin
- Low levels of the brain chemical beta-endorphin

Let's take a look at each component separately.

Volatile Blood Sugar

When you eat carbohydrates (sugars and starches), the glucose (a type of sugar) in your blood increases. Typically, as it rises, your body releases the hormone insulin, which then signals the cells to open up and accept the glucose to be burned as fuel. At best, the system works within a specific range. You eat, your blood sugar rises, insulin is released, the sugar in your blood drops, you get hungry, and you eat again.

Some people are carbohydrate sensitive.[1,2] Their blood sugar goes up more rapidly, they release extra insulin, and consequently their blood sugar drops more quickly. The blood sugar system doesn't work for them. The slope of their blood sugar action is steeper than a normal person's. I believe that carbohydrate sensitivity is one of the hallmarks of sugar sensitivity.

This blood sugar pattern of sugar or carbohydrate sensitivity is not the same as hypoglycemia. Hypoglycemia refers to low blood sugar that occurs when the level of glucose drops below normal and the person experiences fatigue, shakiness, and mental fog. This may be a function of too much insulin or too little food. A sugar sensitive's blood sugar may or may not drop to an abnormally low level. You can be carbohydrate sensitive without being hypoglycemic.

What is important for you is the slope of the blood sugar curve—a faster rise and fall. The blood sugar volatility affects your moods in a big way. When blood sugar rises, you feel great; when it falls, you get really cranky. Blood sugar volatility is the first part of sugar sensitivity.

Serotonin

The second part of sugar sensitivity is a low level of the brain chemical called serotonin or 5HT. Serotonin is a neurotransmitter responsible for mood. Too little of it is associated with depression and impulsivity.[3] Too little and you may have a hard time getting out of bed, getting organized, feeling like you can face the day, creating and fulfilling goals, or feeling that life is worth living.

Serotonin also acts as the brakes in your brain. Think of serotonin as the "just say no" chemical. If you have too little, you may have all the good intentions in the world, but chocolate chip cookies will hop into your mouth before you know it. You may feel you have no self-discipline or no willpower. This is *not* a character flaw; it is biochemical and comes from low serotonin.

Low serotonin is also associated with obsessive and compulsive behaviors.[4] Your brain can "lock" on a task or idea. The brakes get stuck. You munch on a problem over and over, or you get lost in a task and "wake up" five hours later. It is as if your "pay attention" switch is either on or off; there is not a whole lot of flow from one to the other.

Beta-Endorphin

The third part of sugar sensitivity comes from having low levels of the brain chemical called beta-endorphin. Beta-endorphin is a painkiller. It is a survival chemical. It protects you from the pain of running away when a tiger is chasing you. It helps you avoid passing out from the pain when you smash your finger in the car door. Beta-endorphin creates a kind of euphoria. What we call a runner's high is actually a flood of beta-endorphin.

If you have low levels of beta-endorphin, you will have a low tolerance for pain. You won't like going to the dentist. If you fall and skin your knee, it will hurt more. Because beta-endorphin also affects emotional pain, if you are low in this chemical you feel more deeply and are often thought of as being sensitive.

Low levels of beta-endorphin are associated with feeling isolated, inadequate, and helpless.[5] Low levels of beta-endorphin create changes in your brain that make you respond more intensely to the drugs and chemicals that evoke beta-endorphin. You get a bigger high from alcohol.[6] And you respond to sugar as though it were a drug. Sugar evokes beta-endorphin.[7] Your brain likes the effect and is drawn to wanting more. When you use sugar, you feel confident, soothed, and able to cope. You feel attractive and hopeful—until it wears off. And then you need more. Over time the druglike effect diminishes, your tolerance for sugar increases, and you need more and more to achieve the same soothing or energetic effect. *Your addiction to sugar is physiologically real,* and like any addiction, it causes physical and psychological havoc in your life.

I often use the image of a three-legged stool to explain the concept of sugar sensitivity. Each of the biochemical parts forms one of the legs and supports the concept of sugar sensitivity itself, which is the seat of the stool. Each leg as described in the preceding section is well documented in the scientific literature, but the top that connects them all is a new idea.[8] The lived experience and testimony of thousands and thousands of people who now identify themselves as sugar sensitives suggest that I am on to something here.

Not every sugar addict has a problem with all three legs. You may have very low serotonin, reasonably stable blood sugar, and moderately low beta-endorphin. Or you may have extremely low beta-endorphin, moderately low serotonin, and close to normal blood sugar. Or you may have highly reactive blood sugar, low serotonin, and normal beta-endorphin. If all three are a problem, you are in big trouble. Take a look at the symptoms that come with low levels of each of the three and see if you can get a feel for which leg or legs are out of kilter in your sugar-sensitive stool.

LOW BLOOD SUGAR	LOW LEVEL OF SEROTONIN	LOW LEVEL OF BETA-ENDORPHIN
Tired all the time	Depressed	Having low pain tolerance
Tired for no reason	Impulsive	Tearful
Restless and edgy	Short attention span	Experiencing low self-esteem
Confused	Scattered	Feeling sensitive to criticism
Forgetful	Quick to anger	Feeling isolated and inadequate
Inattentive	Aggressive	Seeking crisis
Feeling easily frustrated	Reactive	Feeling "done to" by others
Cranky	Craving sweets	Craving sugar and fat
Short-fused	Craving carbohydrates	Feeling overwhelmed

Traditionally, the medical profession has treated two of the legs of the stool—low blood sugar and low serotonin—as separate problems. The solution for low blood sugar has been to eat regularly and to avoid foods such as sugars and refined carbohydrates. The solution for low serotonin has been to take antidepressants. These medications can work wonders, but they have side effects, take many weeks to start working, and may become less effective after a few months. Finding the right antidepressant for your body and mind may take a great deal of trial and error, which can be a depressing process in and of itself.

The medical profession has not offered a solution for low beta-endorphin. Indeed, low beta-endorphin has not been recognized as a legitimate concern until very recently.

Because there has been so little public discussion about the role of beta-endorphin in well-being, most people with low beta-endorphin have simply intuitively drifted toward the things that make them feel better in the short run, not realizing that they have been self-treating low beta-endorphin. The most common "homemade" or intuitive solutions people have used to raise their beta-endorphin are alcohol, drugs, sugar, fats, compulsive exercise or work, sex, gambling, thrill seeking, and stress. With any of these solutions, you do feel better temporarily. Your confidence goes up, the emotional pain goes away, and you feel less isolated—until the druglike effect wears off. And then you feel worse. So you have to go back for more. The beta-endorphin effect sets you up for an addictive relationship to the things that raise beta-endorphin. You will do anything for even five minutes of relief. You get into a cycle, and you do not know how to get out. In fact, until reading this book, you may not even have understood what is happening in your body or whether there is any other way to be.

If you are sugar sensitive, you may struggle with the whole package. If you are sugar sensitive and overweight, you may have decided that losing weight will fix all the problems. You don't know that your lack of confidence and low self-esteem are a function of your <u>chemistry</u> and <u>*not*</u> of your weight. You think if you just lose weight, you will be okay.

Or you may know that you are depressed, so you start taking an antidepressant. You do feel better, but not in the way you had hoped. You still struggle with feeling inadequate, and you still have times of feeling so tired that you cannot function. Your house stays cluttered, and you still yell at your kids. And you are still fat, sometimes even more so. You now get headaches and can't have an orgasm. The price for getting rid of the depression is high. You still believe if you could just find the right diet, you would lose weight and things would be okay.

This is not how it works. It hasn't worked in the past, and it won't work now. No medication, no amount of willpower, and no weight loss *alone* will resolve the biochemical problem. It is time to address all three biochemical legs of the sugar sensitivity stool.

Your Last Diet! goes right to the heart of all three problems. It is a simple food plan with a powerful impact. "Doing the food"—as I call it—in this plan treats all three biochemical conditions at once in a natural and effective way. Doing the food gives each leg what it needs. You don't have to think separately about your blood sugar, about finding the exact combination for your serotonin, or about fixing your beta-endorphin. You simply do the food, and your body chemistry heals. Look at the kinds of changes in the chart below that happen as you get balanced. I call this kind of balance *radiance*. It is a realistic

map of what you can attain as part of your recovery—
physical, mental, and emotional radiance.

OPTIMAL BLOOD SUGAR	OPTIMAL LEVEL OF SEROTONIN	OPTIMAL LEVEL OF BETA-ENDORPHIN
High energy	Hopeful	Tolerating physical and emotional pain
Appropriate fatigue	Reflective	Sensitive, sympathetic
Relaxed	Able to concentrate	Experiencing high self-esteem
Clear	Creative	Compassionate
Remembers facts	Plans strategically	Connected and in touch
Focused	Cooperative	Hopeful, optimistic
Effective problem solving	Responsive	Taking personal responsibility
Humorous	Engaged	Seeking healthy beta-endorphin-raising activities
Even-tempered	Seeking good health	Solution-oriented

Radiance is a real state that you can have even before
your weight loss if you do the food. Rather than being
foggy, depressed, reactive, impulsive, overwhelmed, and
tired while you're trying to make difficult behavioral
changes, you will be clear, intentional, humorous, and directed. When you are radiant, the chances of your diet
working and lasting go up astronomically. So the first
phase of *Your Last Diet!* is focused on getting you to this

place of radiance. This focus shifts you out of the obsession with the scale into a dynamic and proactive relationship with your healing. It changes everything. It gives you hope, humor, and a sense of possibility. It empowers you down into your cells and bones. Are you not ready for this shift?

"Bake someone happy"—that has always been my motto as long as I can remember.

I grew up knowing that food equals love. As time went on, it became apparent to me that food made me happy, too. Especially chocolate! By the time I was in my twenties I was consuming several candy bars daily. I would buy three bags of miniature Snickers. Would freeze all three, well, I mean I would hide two bags, under some frozen meat, and have the other bag in plain sight so I could get to it easily.

One day, after a huge chocolate binge, I started to feel that my life was not worth living. For the next several weeks I went into a severe, dark depression. One day I decided I had to do something. I was not even functioning, only existing.

Then, after a while, no amount of sugar made me feel happy. All I could do was cry. I was so angry that I couldn't be like other people and eat anything I wanted. Then I began *Your Last Diet!* on www.radiantrecovery.com. For the first time in my life I felt like I was home. I began to understand that I was addicted to sugar.

I have been doing this plan for six months. I have learned to listen to my body, to eat the best kind of foods for me, and to eat at a regular time. I don't feel those pangs of guilt and shame anymore. I have also lost fifty-two pounds since I started. To me, the weight is a bonus. The real present is how great I feel, emotionally and physically,

dured a lifetime of being fat and didn't want the same for me. Now, forty-two years later, after hundreds of diets, I was fatter than ever. I was demoralized, depressed, a hundred pounds overweight. When I looked in the mirror I saw a fat, stupid failure of a woman who would be better off dead. My siblings (all fat), who, like me, were sliding headlong into middle age, were being diagnosed one by one with diabetes, heart disease, and so on, and I was terrified I would be next. My parents had both died in their early fifties of complications from these conditions, and in my late forties I was frozen with fear. In fact, panic was taking over my life, but I still couldn't stop overeating.

Exactly 175 days ago I found *Your Last Diet!* To say it changed my life would be an understatement. It probably *saved* it.

Today I am a different person. I think I am the "real me," which was buried under the self-hatred and fear. I wake up each morning with a sense of positive expectancy, and I go to bed each night feeling a peace inside that had eluded me all of my life. Food no longer rules me. I don't think about it all day long. There is no secret eating, no bingeing, no feelings of being out of control. Just a beautiful, steady, calm, content way of living. I am losing weight and feeling healthy, strong, and self-confident. My panic attacks have stopped. My thinking is clear, and I have so much energy. In fact, now my body tells me it *wants* to exercise! I feel . . . well, there is no other way to put it—positively radiant!

Ruthie

The reason for your weight gain—in fact, anyone's weight gain—is complex and multifactored. The thousands of articles published on obesity attest to this complexity.

Scientists move along inch by inch plotting tiny variables. Some have said obesity is caused by a gene; others, that a pill will make the hunger go away so the weight disappears. No one is giving you the bigger picture about body chemistry and weight gain. No one is helping you make sense of your body so that you can figure out what to do. But *Your Last Diet!* will help.

The Mice Experiments

Let me share some striking information I found buried in the scientific literature. As I looked for scientific evidence to support my theory of sugar sensitivity, I learned that scientists have bred different strains of mice to have certain characteristics. Manipulating the genetic makeup of the mice allows scientists to test more specifically for different components in a problem. Each mouse strain has distinct characteristics. Two strains in particular, the C57 mice and DBA mice, have very different responses to alcohol. The C57 mice are called alcohol-preferring.[9] This means they love alcohol and go back for more and more; if they have a choice between alcohol and water, they will always go for the booze. The DBA mice are called alcohol-avoiding. Booze doesn't call them. They prefer water.

This mouse preference for alcohol is not a learned behavior. The scientists can take a third-generation C57 mouse whose mouse parents never drank, offer it alcohol, and the little C57 will go "Wow! Booze!" the first time it tastes the stuff.[6] And if the scientists do the same with the little DBAs, they will say, "You gotta be kidding me! You want me to drink *that?*" These mice are displaying inherited preferences. Inherited preference for what to drink has a lot to teach us sugar-sensitive people.

In fact, the C57s and DBAs respond the same way to sugars as they do to alcohol. The C57s want more. Let them have something sweet and they will do anything to keep having it.[10] Not only do they love sweet drinks and foods, but they like more concentrated sugars a whole lot more than diluted ones, and they will work hard to get their supply. In fact, when the little C57s have an opportunity to go after sugars, they will sort of forget the other things in life. I think of the C57s as little mouse sugar addicts.

Mind you, these are mouse studies, not people studies. Although there are differences between human biochemistry and mouse biochemistry, I have found that studying the C57 mice is helpful in making sense of why some people respond to sugars, fats, and alcohol so differently.

C57 Characteristics

Let's look a little more at this strain of C57 mice. C57s have lower levels of beta-endorphin, just like us sugar sensitives.[11] Beta-endorphin is the body's natural painkiller, so C57 mice feel pain sooner and more deeply than other mice with higher levels of beta-endorphin. Not only do they feel physical pain more intensely, they also feel emotional pain more intensely. Of course, scientists measure mouse emotional pain a little differently than they would human emotional pain. The C57 mice get upset about being alone. The babies cry a lot when they are taken away from their mothers.[12] The adult C57s respond to stress differently. They crouch in the corner when faced with new, unfamiliar challenges and tests. Scientists believe there is a correlation between these behavioral responses to fear, pain, and uncertainty and the levels of beta-endorphin in the mice's brains.[13] Lower levels of beta-endorphin create these problems.

The brains of the C57 mice work to compensate for the low levels of beta-endorphin by opening up more receptors to try to grab all the beta-endorphin there is. This opening up of extra receptors is called beta-endorphin upregulation. This upregulation allows the C57 mice to experience a more normal response even though they are producing less of the chemicals. But upregulation creates an interesting problem. It is designed to deal with the day-to-day flow of beta-endorphin in the little mouse brain. If a C57 mouse takes something that adds an extra push of beta-endorphin, it will get a bigger reaction because there are now more receptor sites. Things such as alcohol, sugar, and fat evoke beta-endorphin and create a more intense response in the C57 mouse brain.

It is this more intense beta-endorphin response to the effects of alcohol, sugar, and fat that hook the little mouse into wanting more and more. It is a critical factor in creating the addictive response. The scientific data about the differences between the C57 and DBA mice helped me to construct my hypothesis about sugar sensitivity. There is no getting around how uncanny the correlation seems to be in applying the scientific ideas about mice to our lived experience. The science of the C57 mice is actually comforting and instructive for us sugar sensitives as we try to make sense out of what seems to be an irrational attachment to sugar, alcohol, and fat.

There are other differences between the C57 mice and their DBA buddies that can shed light on why sugar-sensitive people so often struggle with their weight. Let me share some of these intriguing C57 characteristics and talk with you about what this might mean for your weight problems.

- C57s are prone to obesity, diabetes, and hypertension.[14]
- C57s gain a disproportionate amount of weight on a high-fat diet. If the DBAs (non-sugar-sensitive mice) and the C57s eat the same number of calories that include a high percentage of calories from fat, the C57s will gain a lot more weight than the DBAs.[14]
- C57s have a different insulin response than the DBA mice. Insulin is the hormone that tells the body to take sugar out of the blood and put it in the cells to be used for fuel. The C57 insulin mechanism doesn't work as well as the DBA one. More sugar stays in the blood and is likely to be stored as fat rather than being burned for energy.[15,16]
- C57s are genetically predisposed to accumulate fat in the stomach area.[17,18]
- C57 mice release more sugar from the liver in response to stress.[19]
- C57s produce less of the hormone leptin in response to eating fat. Leptin shuts off appetite and tells the body to burn fat.[20]
- C57s that exercised more than DBAs while both were on a high-fat diet *still* gained more weight.[21]
- C57s had lower levels of the enzymes sucrase and lipase. They do not digest sugars in the same way as DBAs and so store more.[14]

Science spends billions of dollars on obesity research trying to find out why you are fat and what can be done about it. The insulin scientists work diligently to make sense of the insulin mechanisms, and other scientists grapple with hormonal complexity, yet no one has connected the C57 dots to create a picture of sugar sensitivity to show that this is shared by humans. Before publishing my theories, I talked to my brother, who is a highly respected doctor and CEO of a pharmaceutical company. I asked him whether I should wait for ironclad scientific proof before publishing my first book. He said, "For goodness' sake, you have something that *works*! Get it out there! You are on to something; don't wait for us to catch up."

Even though it may be years before an absolute connection between the two species is proven beyond all scientific doubt, I and others have used the mouse story to create a powerful solution to our weight problem.

Here is a more detailed look at the characteristics and health problems of sugar-sensitive mice:

• *C57s are prone to obesity, diabetes, and hypertension.* C57s get fat, and subsequently develop diabetes and hypertension disproportionately to their non-sugar-sensitive friends. They are genetically predisposed to these conditions. When we read about the idea that some people are more likely than others to get fat or to develop diabetes or hypertension, it makes sense. But let's play with the C57 idea and see what it might mean if we thought of a sugar-sensitive person as a big C57 mouse.

You were hardwired to be fat at birth. You inherited your body from your parents. Before you even started eating differently, your body was waiting to be fat. If no one ever told you this, you may have lived your whole life feeling guilty. You may have thought your weight was a flaw in your personality, not your body. You felt that *you* got this way because of how you ate. *You* were out of control. *You* caused it, and by golly, *you'd* better fix it. These very strong messages may have come from your parents. They certainly come from our culture.

These self-criticisms and judgments by others have been a very painful burden, especially since you have tried and tried to lose weight. Knowing that you have a body that is hardwired toward being fat, like those of the C57 mice, can help you see what you need to do for yourself. *Your Last Diet!* is the solution you need.

• *C57s gained more weight on a high-fat diet than DBA mice on the same diet.* In a study of how increasing consumption of fats would affect weight gain, scientists gave the DBAs (non-sugar-sensitive mice) and the C57s the same number of calories of high-fat mouse chow. On the same number of calories, the C57s gained a lot more weight than their DBA friends did. Think about that! The C57s gained *more* weight on the high-fat diets. It wasn't simply the number of calories they ate that made them gain weight. Something else was going on. When I first read this, the hair on the back of my neck stood up. I *knew* the truth of this in my own body. I knew that I ate less and gained more. I knew that my body responded differently to food. But I had never, ever read anything that said that my intuition was on target.

• *C57s have a different insulin response to sugars than the DBA mice.* C57s are carbohydrate sensitive. Their blood sugar rises more rapidly in response to sugar, and their bodies produce more insulin as a result of this. C57s have an additional problem, called an impaired second-phase insulin response. When the insulin is supposed to be getting the sugar in the blood into the cells, the mechanism doesn't work as well as it should. The C57s are insulin resistant.

More sugar stays in the blood, but the body needs to get rid of it, so it stores the extra as fat. Insulin resistance is one more piece of the fat puzzle. If your sugar-sensitive body really does respond like a C57 mouse, you will be more likely to store fat rather than burn it.

• *C57s are genetically predisposed to accumulate fat in the stomach area.* This particular finding made me laugh. I thought tummy tubby or my aging body shape was a function of genes. I had no idea it might be connected to being sugar sensitive. Somehow, I take great comfort in the idea of the little sugar-loving, alcoholic C57 mice getting fatter in the stomach.

• *C57s respond to stress more intensely.* The body releases sugar (in the form of glycogen) from the liver in response to stress. This response is intended to provide fuel to allow running away in the face of danger. The C57 mice get a bigger release of sugar as glycogen from the liver in response to stress than their lean buddies. This reaction was even more exaggerated in fat C57s.

What might this mean for the sugar-sensitive human? It may mean that stress contributes to your being fat. More stress means more sugar is being released from your own body. If you are not able to process it or metabolize it adequately, it will be stored as fat. In addition, since you have a more pronounced reaction to the sugar, you may grow to depend on the stress-induced sugar "hit." You may seek out stressful situations in order to get a sugar rush.

• *C57s do not produce the hormone leptin in response to fat intake the same way that non-sugar-sensitive mice do.* Leptin, which shuts off appetite and tells the body to burn fat, seems to be another of the genetically wired contributors to fat levels. Leptin tells the body how much fat is stored. When it says, "Enough," the body knows to eat less and turn up the fat-burning process. If C57s have lower levels of leptin, this may be true for sugar-sensitive people as well. Think of what this may mean for you. Rather than getting a leptin message to burn fat, you sit around getting fatter and fatter.

• *C57s exercised more than DBAs while both were on a high-fat diet and still gained more weight.* C57s develop severe obesity when placed on high-fat diets. Researchers at Duke University wanted to see if exercise would affect how much weight the C57s gained compared to the other strain of mice. They put both strains of mice on a high-fat diet. As expected, the C57s gained more weight without consuming more calories. But to the amazement of the researchers, the C57s actually exercised more than their lean friends did. The researchers officially state that "diet-induced obesity is not explainable by reduced levels of physical activity."

This researcher language may mean that you are not necessarily a couch potato if you are overweight. Being fat is generally blamed on your lack of exercise. You may exercise a lot and still not be able to figure out why you do not lose weight. The findings about the C57 mice and exercise suggest that there is far more to losing weight than what you have been told and what is typically known.

• *C57s had lower levels of the enzymes sucrase and lipase. They do not digest fats and sugars in the same way as DBAs.* Researchers found that the little C57s had lower levels of the intestinal enzymes sucrase and lipase when their diets were high in sugar. So C57s don't digest sugar and fat in the same way that the little lean mice do. If sugars and fats are not digested properly, they cannot be used as fuel. They stay in the bloodstream and get converted to fat.

Put all these pieces together, and you get a tubby little mouse who has a hard time losing weight and is prone to diabetes and hypertension. If the C57 obesity research reveals biochemical truths that apply to us sugar-sensitive people, it certainly helps to explain why you gain more weight and why you have a harder time losing weight than your normal friends do.

C57s and Beta-endorphin

The C57 profile has many other interesting pieces that can help you make sense of why you are the way you are. Let's look at the brain chemistry of the little C57 mice. As I said earlier, C57s inherit lower levels of the brain chemical called beta-endorphin. Lower levels mean a brain adjustment to create more beta-endorphin sites. More beta-endorphin sites mean a bigger "hit" in response to things that produce beta-endorphin, such as sugar and alcohol. This contributes to the C57s really liking sugar and alcohol and wanting more. It is why C57s are called alcohol-preferring mice.

Beta-endorphin withdrawal is responsible for cravings. When the beta-endorphin effect of alcohol or sugar wear off, the empty beta-endorphin receptors scream for more. With more beta-endorphin receptor sites screaming, you will have bigger cravings than the person who has a normal brain. People who are alcoholic generally have lower

levels of beta-endorphin than those who are not alcoholic. Because the low levels of beta-endorphin are geneti- ←
cally determined, the sons, daughters, and grandchildren
of alcoholics may inherit these lower levels and thus may
be more at risk for alcoholism.

This same inherited brain chemistry also affects cravings for sweet and high-fat foods. I consider it a key part
of sugar sensitivity. You are born with a bigger reaction to
beta-endorphin. Sugars and fats evoke beta-endorphin. Because of your brain chemistry, you get a bigger "hit" from
the sweet and fat foods, so you become physiologically—
not just psychologically or emotionally—addicted to them.

Sugar Sensitivity and Serotonin

C57 mice also have lower levels of another brain chemical
called serotonin. I believe that these lower levels of serotonin are a key factor in sugar sensitivity in mice and humans. For instance, serotonin regulates mood and the
ability to say no (impulse control) in humans. Serotonin
provides the brain's brakes. If you have low levels of it, you
will be impulsive and reactive. You will shoot your mouth
off at the wrong times. You will say, "I am not going to eat
any more cookies," and then eat the whole bag. You will
insist that a new diet is "it" and then three weeks later give
up and forget it. You will wake up in the middle of Febru-
ary and feel that you cannot function another day. This is
all because of low serotonin.

What and when you eat affects serotonin levels. When
you diet, you reduce the levels of serotonin in your brain.
Dieting actually makes you less able to say no and more
vulnerable to depression. This is one reason traditional
diets do not work for sugar sensitives. You feel much

worse than other people on a diet. This shift in serotonin levels doesn't happen overnight, however. It takes a couple of weeks. But the low serotonin creeps up on you and whacks you in the head about four to five weeks into the latest diet.

Your serotonin levels are related to the insulin levels in your blood. Many diets are designed to minimize insulin levels by reducing foods that evoke insulin. While this is good for your overall health and for reducing your insulin resistance, it zaps your serotonin levels. You can feel terrific on one of those diets for the first few weeks, and then *pow*—you feel as if you can't do it another day, and a slice of bread sets you off on a three-week binge. This is the effect of low serotonin.

Because serotonin is the brain chemical that helps you say no, whenever you minimize your insulin levels, you will be less and less able to stick with the diet. And you will get more and more depressed as the lowered serotonin contributes to a bleaker mood.

What to Do with This Information

This information about brain chemicals and mice does not mean that being sugar sensitive is a hopeless condition. You *can* fix it. You may feel that you are destined to be fat no matter what, *but these feelings of hopelessness come from your biochemistry.* And you *can* change the feelings *and* your biochemistry.

Your Last Diet! will help get you a kind of DBA energy— a hopeful, confident, goal-setting energy—by healing your sugar sensitivity. You will become more able to solve the problem of your weight rather than feel defeated by it. *Your Last Diet!* will help to compensate for your C57-like

sugar-sensitive wiring. It won't be fast, but it will be certain. The plan isn't going to fix every single one of your problems, but it will give you the emotional and physical stability to allow you to use all the life skills and resources you have developed over the years to address your other problems. *Your Last Diet!* has already done this for thousands of other sugar sensitives. In this book and on our community website at www.radiantrecovery.com, they attest to its effectiveness for sugar-sensitive people.

Let's go back and review what you have learned so far. ←
If you are sugar sensitive, you have a body that acts like a big C57 mouse. You respond differently to sugars and fats, you gain weight disproportionately, you don't rise to new challenges well or confidently, you have a hard time saying no, and you struggle with an addictive relationship with sweets and white foods.

What and how you eat has a profound effect on your body. Because of the sugar-sensitive body chemistry, you are naturally drawn to a high-sugar, high-carbohydrate, high-fat diet. These kinds of foods increase your beta-endorphin levels and enhance your serotonin levels in the short term. They comfort you and make you feel satisfied— as if you are coping. But what you think is comforting you is actually creating the problem of mood swings and weight gain. Putting a high-sugar, high-fat, high-carbohydrate diet into a C57 metabolism is a recipe for disaster.

In many ways you have been a sitting duck for a weight problem. Your biochemistry makes you vulnerable to gaining more and more weight. You become depressed and impulsive. You try lots of different ways to lose weight, but your weight keeps going up despite your best intentions. This pattern is devastating. After years of spinning like a hamster on a wheel, you have come to feel hopeless.

Your Last Diet! helps you change this. Changing what and when you eat will shift your sugar-sensitive body chemistry. Your moods will become stable. You will be able to follow through on your intentions, and you will lose weight. Permanently. You will heal the shame and feel hopeful, optimistic, and radiant.

If you are sugar sensitive, losing weight needs to be done in several phases. This is the plan we follow in *Your Last Diet!* First, you change your body chemistry with a food plan that lays the physical and emotional foundation for weight loss. You get steady, and then you develop a weight loss plan that is perfect for your body. Essentially, you first shift your brain and body chemistry from being like that of the C57 mice to being like that of the DBA mice. By doing so, you will be able to lose the weight that the sugar-sensitive chemistry created. Rather than being impulsive, impatient, and reactive as you diet, you will be reflective and effective. Rather than feeling hopeless and overwhelmed, you will feel optimistic and empowered.

The first phase of *Your Last Diet!* will prepare you for dieting and weight loss by:

- Getting your brain stable enough to follow directions
- Increasing your serotonin levels enough to have impulse control and to be able to stick with your intention
- Stopping beta-endorphin spiking so you don't have huge mood swings and cravings resulting from withdrawal
- Increasing your beta-endorphin levels so you feel confident and able to make changes and solve problems

All this will happen before you even think about the scale. *Your Last Diet!* is different from anything you have ever done before. You do most of the work *before* you start

the losing-weight phase. The plan is designed to get you to *stop* thinking about the scale and stop fretting about how many pounds you have to lose before your daughter's wedding. This is a radical departure from what you are used to, but in the long run you *will* lose weight.

Just sit still for a minute. The plan is very simple. All you need to do and everything you need to learn will be explained in simple, straightforward terms. Basically, you simply do the food. You follow the program for healing sugar sensitivity with food. I will teach you what this means. You will take baby steps, follow a very clear sequence, and do the steps as they are outlined. Your body and your brain will change, and you will feel better. Think of this book as a weight loss map for sugar sensitives. You can't get from point A to point B in an instant. But you will always know the way from one to the other, and you won't ever get lost.

Let's get started. I want you to feel the radiance that I have every day.

2

Getting Started

Now that you know about being sugar sensitive and its implications for your weight loss, you may be asking, "Where's the diet?" or "What do I eat?" These questions are part of your old diet mentality. We *will* answer them, but for now please take a deep breath and be open to understanding that a key part of *Your Last Diet!* is changing these old sugar-sensitive thinking patterns. You aren't going to do weight loss yet. First you are going to heal your sugar sensitivity. Your sugar-sensitive brain needs to get focused and steady and have the ability to say no.

No sugar addict has all the C57 characteristics outlined in the last chapter. But most have more than one and usually several. These biochemical characteristics affect your weight and your ability to deal with the world. To be able to sort out what you need to do, how *you* can best lose weight and keep it off, you first need to be in a place of balance. You need to be clear on how your body and brain react to food, you need to learn to control your im-

whole thing today. Ninety-nine percent of the thousands of people who are doing this program with me online start with the same impatience and even desperation. The general, unspoken attitude is "Yeah, right, Kathleen. Great ideas, but you don't understand. I need to deal with the pounds *now*. Then I can do that healing stuff."

Fact is, I *do* understand, way more than you can imagine. I, like you, tried every diet, from the grapefruit and cottage cheese diet of many, many years ago to a hospital plan and all the more recent ones. My highest weight was 265, my lowest 145. My closet had fat clothes and skinny clothes. I knew calories, fat grams, and counting. Every piece you struggle with, I have lived.

If you want one more diet, this is not the story for you. If you want one *last* diet, if you want what we as recovering sugar addicts have—clarity, calm, radiance, and our true weight—then you will have to do what we do. This means doing the steps *in sequence* and doing them slowly. By slowly I do not mean in four weeks or even in eight weeks. This plan is about a lifestyle, a long-term change in the way you relate to your food and your body. For this program to succeed, you have to radically change your mindset and your usual expectations. Essentially, you have to live in the process and give your body enough time to catch up to the willingness you have to change your life. Your body, your cells, and your spirit need to catch up and integrate with your commitment to heal.

Because I have lived this process myself, and because I have shared the process with so many people just like you, I have a great deal of compassion for how hard this is to do. In fact, I think it is almost impossible to do it alone. This is why I developed an online community where people get in touch with other sugar sensitives and share what they are going through every day. They talk with one another all the time, share tips, and give and get help.

You are nor alone on *Your Last Diet!* Every day new people find their way to the online community forum and join the *Your Last Diet!* program. They consistently report that they just started the program and are already on Step 5 after the first week. The old-timers laugh and start repeating our mantra: *slow down.* Over and over and over. And then they tell their stories. They tell stories of healing, of release from compulsion, of feeling transformed, of knowing what to do, and of losing weight.

I know that even after you have started the program, you will immediately want to know what else you can do. You will be saying, "What's next?" Other diets and many doctors have conditioned you to expect the entire set of instructions all at once on day one and to start losing weight right away: Follow this plan, take this drug, reduce your calories, and increase your exercise. Get started, get moving, and be thin. *Your Last Diet!* is a radical departure from this diet tradition. You are going to make some major changes. Think of it as literally rewiring your brain and your body. We want to change the chemistry that makes you impulsive, out of control, and gain weight. We also want to repattern your behavior slowly and over a long period of time so that the biochemical changes and the behavioral patterns match up in a new way.

In fact, the hardest part of *Your Last Diet!* is not even the food part; it is shifting the expectation about what will get you to where you want to be. In my experience and the experience of the thousands of people I have counseled, actually losing the weight is a relatively minor part of the process. It is more like an afterthought rather than the primary purpose. The healing is the biggie. But in our culture, we are brainwashed into believing that if we simply lose weight, everything will be all right. It is so easy to forget that every time you have lost weight you have gained it back. Or you forget the feelings of deprivation, the cost of losing weight. You forget the emotional agony that went along with the diet process. This time around we are going to change all of that.

This is a very difficult concept to grasp. You can't just will it to make sense. You can't just skim the book, nod, agree, and say, "Okay, I'm ready. Where is the diet?" You will actually have to live the doing of it. One day, one choice at a time. Starting *Your Last Diet!* requires a huge leap of faith. Intuitively you will know that this program and these ideas are so right and so on target that they will truly work. But your fat self, the one who has struggled for so long, is going to nudge you with its impatience. That one will whisper in your ear to get moving, go faster, do it all at once, tweak the edges.

You can read ahead if you like. You can think about what is to come. But you have to start by getting your foundation in place solidly. We want this to work.

Our first task is to heal your sugar-sensitive biochemistry. Let's take a look at what is going on for you. As you learned earlier, sugar-sensitive people have three basic imbalances in their systems: volatile blood sugar, low serotonin, and low beta-endorphin. It appears that we can restore these three systems to balance by making some simple changes in your diet. Many of us have suspected a link between our food and our mood. Few have imagined how profound that link is. The seven healing steps that create stability in your body and mind are actually quite simple. They are:

1. Eat breakfast with protein.
2. Keep a food journal to note what you eat and how you feel.
3. Eat three meals a day with protein.
4. Take a specific set of vitamins and have a potato before bed.
5. Shift from white foods to brown foods.
6. Stop using sugars.
7. Enhance your radiance.

The seven steps are simple, but they are not easy. Going through them carefully and attentively can take six to eight months. As you learn each step, you will learn more about an entirely new way of eating and thinking about your body. And you will feel better and be healthier.

You progress through the seven steps and build on the strength of the changes that come out of them. The steps work. They create balance. If you want an extensive tutorial on the steps, read either of my first two books. But at this point, it is time to get started. Let's begin with breakfast.

Step 1: Eat Breakfast with Protein

Have breakfast every day within an hour of getting up. Every day. No skipping. Breakfast should include both protein and some complex carbohydrates. Your body needs protein for a number of things. First of all, protein is the basis of good health. Your body needs protein to produce amino acids that run your body. They build and rebuild cells and repair things that are broken. For sugar-sensitive people, one particular amino acid, tryptophan, is particularly critical. Tryptophan is the raw material that your body uses to make serotonin. Without sufficient raw material from tryptophan, your serotonin factory can't make what you need. Protein supplies the tryptophan that is the raw material.

This is *not* a high-protein plan. It is a regular and consistent moderate-protein plan. How much protein is enough for each meal? There are basically two ways to decide. You can use either the counting method or the looking method. In the looking method you use your fist as a guideline: Have a fist-sized portion of protein at each meal. Obviously, if you weigh more or have a bigger fist, you will need to eat more protein. The fist-sized portion applies to protein that you can actually hold in your hand. So milk wouldn't count as a good meal protein. Cottage cheese does because it is denser.

Many people prefer the counting method, particularly when they are starting to work on the program, because they feel more confident that they are getting the right amount of protein they need. If you divide your total body weight in half, you will get the approximate number of grams of protein you should have per day. For example if you weigh 150 pounds, you should have about 75 grams of protein a day. Divide the result by three to find out how much protein you should have at each meal. So a 150-pound person should have approximately 25 grams of protein at each meal.

If you are a very large person (over 250 pounds), you will want to have *less* than this because the ratio of your body fat to your lean muscle mass is so much higher. We are looking to ensure that your muscles and brain have the protein they need to function, not to give you extra fat. Ideally, you would calculate your body mass index and construct a proportion-of-protein table suited to your actual weight. That seems a little unrealistic unless you are working with a nutritionist, trainer, or health care professional who can do it for you. I suggest you simply use 250 pounds as a base to calculate your protein needs if you weigh more than that. It should work well for you. If it doesn't, add a little more protein.

Many people ask me how to convert grams of protein into ounces of food. This is actually a complicated question and not an easy one to know off the top of your head. You cannot simply say, "Oh, there are *x* grams in an ounce," because actual protein food is made up of protein and fat and water and sometimes carbohydrates. To figure out how many grams of protein are in foods, you will need to get a protein gram list. You can find one at a bookstore, or you can go online and find a nutrition program that calculates protein grams. To get you started, here is a list of breakfast foods with their protein content.[22]

Cheddar cheese, 3.4 oz	25
2 T protein powder	24
Sliced turkey, 4 oz	20
3 eggs	19
Sausage, 3 links	15–45 (read labels)
Cottage cheese, 4 oz	14
Peanut butter, 2 T	8
Yogurt, 8 oz	8

If your eyes start to glaze over at trying to figure this out, just get simple. Choose the foods that make the most sense for your lifestyle and develop a routine. Many of the people on *Your Last Diet!* make a protein-carb shake for breakfast because it's quick, it's easy, and it supplies the amount of protein needed.

In addition, it is imperative that you have some carbohydrates with your breakfast: oatmeal, whole grain toast, bagels, or muffins are okay. At this stage in the game, you are not yet making changes away from really sweet foods. But if you can, I want you to start paying attention to the foods you are eating. Make sure you are getting enough protein. See which carbohydrates hold you longer and keep you from getting hungry before lunch. You may find a big difference between having oatmeal and having sugared cereal. Most of the folks doing this plan love oatmeal and think it is a wonder food. They even learn to enjoy it without piles of brown sugar!

Here are some sample breakfasts:

1. Poached eggs, sausage, and English muffins
2. Cottage cheese mixed with fresh peaches and a bran muffin
3. Waffles made with nuts and protein powder in the batter and cooked apples on top
4. Oatmeal with cottage cheese and applesauce
5. Cheese omelet with hash browns and tomatoes
6. Beef or chicken burrito
7. Oatmeal with milk or yogurt, fruit, and a side of turkey sausages
8. Two hard-boiled eggs and juice (good to have in the car on the way to work)
9. Bagel with cream cheese piled with lox
10. Corned beef hash and two eggs with a slice of toast

Some of these breakfasts may not have enough protein for your body size. If that is the case, simply adjust them as needed. Most sugar-sensitive people do not eat breakfast when they start the program. This is even more true if they are overweight. They like skipping breakfast because it helps them feel "lean and mean" for a little while. They like the feeling that comes from the first cup of coffee. Some prefer to exercise without eating first, and others feel they simply too busy to think of breakfast. Take the time. You have to eat breakfast with protein as you start the program.

When I talk about breakfasts like these, people new to the program have all sorts of concerns, like "Won't this make me gain weight?" "Isn't this too much cholesterol?" "But those foods have fat!" "I don't think eating red meat is healthy." These questions have come up over and over on our community forum and the *Your Last Diet!* beginner list. So you can feel comforted that you are not alone in having some ambivalence about eating breakfast. In fact, some people take several months to master actually having breakfast every morning, before they learn to love it.

But let me address some of those concerns for you. Eating breakfast will not make you gain weight. It will give your brain what it needs to function. And yes, some of these breakfast foods have fat. You are not doing a low-fat diet. Later on down the road, when you get to the weight loss component of your plan, you will adjust the kind and the amount of fats you eat. When you are starting off, have breakfast with protein and pick foods that you enjoy. If you don't want to eat red meat, you certainly don't have to. If you are concerned about the cholesterol in eggs, choose another alternative. Later on you will learn more about the science of cholesterol and why in fact *Your Last Diet!* may very well reduce your cholesterol levels significantly. For now, simply find a breakfast that works for you.

Often sugar-sensitive people love to skip breakfast. If you don't eat for a long time, your body releases beta-endorphin to protect you from the pain of what it thinks is starvation. When you get up in the morning, you haven't eaten since dinnertime, or at least since your last snack. Not eating breakfast extends the "not eating" time, and your body deals with the stress by releasing beta-endorphin. You feel confident and lean as a result. I called skipping breakfast a "starvation high."

When you start eating breakfast, even though you feel better, part of you misses this confident, lean feeling. You often forget the 10 A.M. crashes that always followed and led to inhaling a sweet roll with your latte or a doughnut with your third cup of coffee. So learning to eat breakfast can be more complicated than it seems at first blush. However, the payoff is tremendous. Once you actually start having a regular breakfast, you will feel a whole lot better right away. Within a week, you will start to notice a difference.

Focusing on breakfast gets you started. It may take some time to master the pattern of breakfast with protein every day. Continue to work on it, and let it become part of your daily pattern. Try to quiet your impatience in waiting to surge ahead. Because you are bringing so much frustration, pain, and desperation to this program, it is perfectly natural to want results now. We have all been there. I want you to have results that last and that heal and transform you. And those kinds of results are going to take time. Mastering breakfast with protein and carbs every day may take weeks, sometimes months.

When people ask me when to move on to the next step, I always say you are ready when you love the step you are on. When you feel that you love having breakfast, that you have a sense of joy and competence on consistency with breakfast, then start thinking about Step 2.

Step 2: Use Your Journal to Record What You Eat and How You Feel

Writing down what and when you eat is crucial. Your food journal is the primary working tool for helping you understand what your body is doing. To be able to design your weight loss plan, you need to be able to know how your own body responds to the foods you eat—how your moods change, when your energy flags, when you are charged up or exhausted and blue. The only way to learn this personal connection between food and mood is writing down what and when you eat and how you feel, every single day. Over time your journal will give you clues about the patterns and concerns relevant to your body. Even if you already kept a journal for another diet or eating plan, do not skip this step. The journal is going to teach you about your sugar-sensitive body. If you skip the journal, you will dilute the effectiveness of the program. Skip the journal and your body will have no way to talk to you.

Resistance to Writing It Down

If you are just starting your food plan, you may not like this idea of doing a food journal. "I don't need to do it" and "I know what I eat" are the words I hear from almost every new client. They just want to make the changes to their food and really can't be bothered to go to the trouble of writing it down. These feelings are legitimate. If you have never really had a payback from doing the work of a food journal, it becomes a bother. But this time it's different. This food journal is going to teach you surprising new things about your body, things that will help you balance your emotions and lose weight once and for all.

four columns, you can easily see the connection between what you eat and how you feel physically and emotionally. Opposite is an example of what a blank page of a food journal might look like.

Start by jotting down what you eat and when you eat it. Be specific with the amounts of what you are having. Rather than write down "chicken and vegetables for dinner," for instance, write that you had a medium-size piece of broiled chicken breast, 1 cup of green beans, and 1 baked potato with butter.

Try to write in your journal as you go through the day. Carry your journal with you. If you can't keep your journal with you, take notes and then transcribe them in the evening. If you forget to write in your journal, put in the day and time anyhow and write that you don't remember what you had. If you remember how you feel but not what you ate, write that down. *Not* remembering is significant information—sort of like standing up a date. Write down that you don't remember, too!

Physical feelings can show you that your body is out of sorts. First you will notice your body's "comment" (stomachache, fatigue, etc.), and then you will learn to interpret what it means. Some people have a hard time doing their food journal because they honestly do not know how they feel. They get discouraged because all they are doing is writing "fine" or "okay," or sometimes "horrible" or "discouraged." Learning to recognize the subtlety of what your body has to say may take some time, because you are literally learning a new language. You are going to have to practice to become fluent in body talk. For now, simply make a commitment to keeping the journal carefully. Over time you will become more and more skilled in using it. If you don't have a journal, you have no record of your process. If you don't keep a journal, your body has no way to talk to you.

You may find that you really do not like the idea of the journal. You just cannot bring yourself to do it. Or you try and try to keep it up, but you don't. It is possible to develop a relationship to your resistant feelings and understand them better. Use your journal to see where and how these feelings work in your life. Because you have been eating breakfast every day and your brain and body are less foggy, you can now learn more about where and how your resistance works.

I developed a wonderful exercise to deal with my own resistance. I thought that trying to break it would only make it stronger. So I imagined the part of me that was resisting the journal. It was the part that did not want to see what I was eating. She had huge shame about being fat. She believed the messages that it was her fault that I had gained weight. She did not want to look at the facts. So I decided to be tender and nonjudgmental to help her feel safe. I imagined she was a real person, and I invited her in to dialogue with me. I gave her a voice and pretended she could answer. It was as if we went out for tea. I explained that I needed to be able to learn about my body, and if she sabotaged the process, I wouldn't get very far. I asked her to help me understand what she was afraid of.

I talked to my resistance about where I wanted to go with the next phase of my plan. By taking manageable baby steps, I kept her from spooking and blocking my journal. As I went through this exercise, humor served me well. "Okay, my dear, we are going to do a little more detailed food journaling. How about we put the notes right here in the ol' margin. . . . Too boring? You know this already? Naw, let's go deeper with it. Let's start looking at some of the things you don't really want to see."

This exercise gave me a way to give my resistance a personal voice and to connect with the message it had for me.

I have had that sabotaging voice since I was little. I like to push limits—to see how much can I get away with. My parents called it stubbornness; I called it obstinacy. It even exists independently in my body in my left leg. If I get to feeling stubborn enough, my left leg will stomp. It has since I was little. (My mother would say, "Don't you stomp your leg at me!") I learned to laugh at this one night many years ago, while lying in bed with my husband. We were having an argument, and while actually lying down—not standing, mind you—my leg stomped . . . on nothing! We laughed so hard!

Well, that is when I realized how obstinate I am with rules, or anytime someone tells me what I have to do. That's why whenever I went on a diet I would rebel and get angry. For a while I waited for that to happen here, but it hasn't. The biochemistry of my left leg is healing, and so much of this program depends on my finding out what is good for me. The journal is key.

When Kathleen says, "Love your resistant voices," it is good advice. That is what I have done through my journal, and now I hardly hear from them. My left leg hasn't stomped in a long time!

Stephanie

Find what works for you. Get creative. This is an important part of your process. Notice you are going slowly here. You aren't trying to get your resistance to go faster. You aren't being sly or trying to fool it. You aren't trying to break it. Breaking things down never works. Your denial has kept you safe and allowed you to live your life— perhaps not well, but you have managed. It has been a survival method for you. You are just being clear about the fact that yes, you are going to move to the next step (that part is not negotiable) and you really want the resistant part's help. Treasure your resistance. Bless it. Learn from it. Remember, resistance is a gift.

Let me give you a specific example of how your journal can help you do the plan. I have been journaling for many years. At one point I noticed that I wasn't including what I drank during the day in my journal. I was flirting with drinking Diet Coke, but on some level I knew this wasn't a good thing for me—normally I don't use caffeine and try to avoid aspartame—so I conveniently stopped writing about it in my journal. Rather than beating myself up, I started laughing at both my resistance and my denial. As I recorded the Diet Coke, I saw that I was becoming more tired and cranky, which of course reinforced my need for the "drug." In my denial, I had convinced myself it was the thing that relieved the bad feelings—a true addictive response! The very thing I thought was solving the problem was actually creating it. Putting this in my journal changed the pattern. I stopped drinking the Diet Coke soon after.

The day after I stopped drinking Diet Coke, I experienced a level of darkness and depression I could never have imagined. I don't tend to be depressed, but that day my arms and legs felt like lead and the world looked black. I thought that if I had to live this way all the time, I wouldn't do it. The darkness was so big and so spooky that it really shook me. So, being a true and incurable addict, I went and got my "drug." And *bam*—within ten minutes I felt just fine. Let me tell you, that got my attention big-time.

The day after I stopped the Diet Coke, I knew how I was going to feel, I knew what was causing it, and I simply walked through it and wrote it down. My journal reminded me there was an absolute, direct connection between my feelings and what I had had to drink the day before. Connection to your body is what you are seeking in your food journal in this first stage of your healing. And as you are getting ready for the weight loss phase of your plan, the journal becomes even more crucial.

Using Your Food Journal as a Tool for Discovery

Let's take a look at how the journal can serve *you*. Once you have recorded several days' worth of food and feelings in your journal, you will discover what a great tool a journal can be for detecting the roots of your moods and behaviors. For example, you may slip off the food plan and find yourself upset about the piece of chocolate cake that jumped into your mouth. You cite the day you ate the cake as the day your slip began, but go through the pages of your journal to see what other things led up to the day with the cake. You may find you had a glass of wine two days before and a scone with your latte the day before the cake. Slippage is usually gradual. It creeps in with choices that are easy to forget. Your journal will help you track how you are doing.

Get a yellow marker. Now look at the three days before the chocolate cake. Highlight all the "just a" events, the times when you had "just a" little piece of a cookie, or "just a" piece of French bread, or "just a" tiny free sample of a new brand of pizza at the supermarket.

Each "just a" is a step up the ladder that leads to the top of the biochemical slide, which leads to slipping and release. The chocolate cake may be the big, attention-getting, undeniable whoosh down the slide, but it is the end of the slip, not the beginning. If you don't keep a food journal to document what you are eating and when, you will never, ever see this. Highlighting the "just a" events in yellow will enable you to understand what the steps were that set you up for sliding off your program. If you write things down, you can see when you are starting the process; you can note the tiny little steps and make changes before you get into bigger trouble.

Using Your Food Journal to Know Your Progress

Your food journal also provides a marker for your progress. When you look back, your early journals will seem very different from your later ones. Your way of doing the food will get clearer and more focused. You will start to see that the days you feel off are the days your food is off. All these years when you felt off, you may have felt it was because of the stress on the job, or PMS, or your kids' demands, or being overweight. Not so. It was from having a sugar-sensitive biochemistry. Your food journal will show you how closely your food affects how you feel. When your food is wobbly, your life will be wobbly.

The relationship between food and quality of life is powerful. You cannot possibly imagine how powerful before you start a food journal. The cornerstone of your healing, your food journal, is also the first step in creating a relationship with your body.

I wish there was a magic formula to tell you how long it takes, but alas, there isn't. It is a gradual process. It just starts with realizing that you could take that dessert or leave it. Then another time you walk by the doughnut shop and realize the glazed crullers just don't sound all that appealing. Finally one day you wake up and realize it has been two and a half years and you haven't had any sugar.

Michelle

It is time for you to move on to the next step, in which you do your journal pretty consistently. Sometimes it takes a while to love your journal. Doing the journal at this stage in the program is hard because you don't like seeing what and how you are eating. Yet that is why it is so important. The journal is a powerful way to get you to acknowledge how things really are. The journal addresses the mental, physical, and emotional impact of your eating. It moves from denial into a clear, nonjudgmental look at how you feel and what you eat.

You do not have to do your journal perfectly. Work on it as best you can. You may find that as your food improves, you will enjoy your journal more. You may start to get a kick out of seeing how things have changed. The journal gives you a sense of history. In the beginning it may be full of words such as "tired," "cranky," and "foggy." As horrible as it is to notice all this in the beginning, it is exciting to see and hear the shift. A few more "I felt clear and focused today" or "Enjoyed taking the kids out to the park today and wasn't impatient." Your energy improves, your headaches diminish, you feel stable.

To be honest, some people skip doing the journal when they start *Your Last Diet!* because they think it's un-necessary. They think they know what they eat. Or they think they eat the same thing every day. Or they simply are not interested in looking at the food. Or they have too many memories of other diet plans that required a log. Or their self-criticisms and judgments are so negative they just can't bear to bring themselves to write or read the journal. So these folks just skip the second step, continue with the other steps, and then hit a wall. They don't feel well; things are not working. They come to the online community forum or the online community support email lists to try to sort it out. The first reply is always "What does your journal say?" With no journal, there is no data, no way to sort things out effectively. It is hit or miss, and the problems cannot get solved easily.

I have been intrigued to see that even the people who start out not doing the journal come back to it. It is such a key part of the program that I encourage you, urge you to do it. I still journal, and I love what it teaches me. I forget what is happening with my food, start feeling cranky, and go back to my journal: "Oh, yeah, forgot to have lunch at noon, and ate at three." If I didn't have a way to find the contributing factors, I would still grope around and at-tribute the feelings to stress or external factors. Please keep your journal.

I think the amazing part of Kathleen's plan is how one step magically leads us to the next and the next. Once the mo-mentum gets rolling toward recovery and radiance, every-thing seems to draw us closer to it. (I mastered a step, and my body seemed to know I was ready for the next step; I found myself drawn to it.)

Sheila

The next step seems pretty straightforward.

Step 3: Eat Three Meals a Day at Regular Intervals, with Protein at Each Meal

This step will stabilize your blood sugar and make sure you have both the amino acids and the other nutrients you need to produce the brain chemicals that are so critical for your sugar-sensitive body. Having three meals a day at regular intervals also creates a significant behavioral change that will serve you well. By starting and stopping a meal three times a day, you are also going to reinforce the behavior of starting and stopping. Most sugar-sensitive people graze throughout the day. Your sugar feelings make you terrified of not having enough and so you eat more than you need, or you get bored and so you eat, or you feel something and think it is hunger and so you eat. Most often what you feel is not hunger but sugar withdrawal. The feeling of edginess and needing something is biochemical, but it is rarely hunger.

By training your body to recognize that it will be fed at regular intervals, you will help it to feel safe. Because it won't have to wonder if there is going to be another meal coming, it will stop thinking that it needs to hold on to whatever you eat since it might never get another chance for fuel. Your body will know that food is coming and will burn the food and fuel it already has.

In Step 1 you learned about how much protein to have at each meal. In this step you are mastering the practice of eating regularly at every meal. Plan the times, plan the food. Have enough protein at each meal, and include some carbohydrates and some good fat, such as olive oil. If you are still having sweet things (which is most likely at this step), continue to have them, but have them *with* your meals. Desserts are fine if you have them *with* the meal. If you are drinking soda, have it with your meal, not in the middle of the afternoon.

You are also going to begin to train your body to stop eating at the end of a meal. Stopping is a big deal for people with low serotonin. Serotonin provides the brakes that control your impulses; low serotonin means bad brakes, and so you are not good at saying no. Stopping helps to reinforce behaviorally the steadiness that you are creating neurochemically.

At this point in your recovery, the part of your sugar-sensitive brain that tells you that you are full does not work very well. The "I am full" switch (called your satiety switch) is related to both your serotonin and leptin levels, which are probably low. Low serotonin means your switch is bad. Over time, as you follow this plan, you are going to repair this switch, but in the meantime, you are going to have to reset the switch manually. By stopping a meal, (finishing rather than grazing), you are training your body to know that finishing a meal means that you stop eating until the next meal.

As you are moving toward having regular meals, you will want to start planning your shopping more carefully. Martha, one of the members of the *Your Last Diet!* community, designed a meal planner for herself. Here is how her planner evolved:

1. When I started, I had no idea what was a protein, what was a healthy carbohydrate, or how to shop. I started with the lists in *Potatoes Not Prozac* and *The Sugar Addict's Total Recovery Program* and went from there. I studied things at the grocery store. The little numbers on the labels helped me get to know how many grams of protein things had. This helped a lot at the beginning to see how different protein foods compared.

2. I decided to make a list of the things I liked, not just someone else's suggestions. So I made up a list for proteins, healthy carbs, and greens and other vegetables.

3. I started using those lists to plan my meals and then used that to help me plan my shopping. I put together a shopping list and incorporated it with my meal planner.

4. I go grocery shopping on Saturday mornings and print out a fresh copy of the planner before I start. Looking at the week ahead, if I have some rush-rush day and need on-the-go food, I plan for it. Or if I have a dinner at a restaurant, I plan for it. For each day, I jot down the basic meal plan. Then I use a yellow highlighter to highlight the foods I need to buy on my grocery shopping trip.

5. I have plenty of space to write all sorts of other things, like if I need light bulbs or toilet paper. It works really well. If I need to go to two different stores for different foods, I might use another color highlighter to show which foods come from a different store.

6. I carry the plan around with me in my appointment book at all times. At the end of the week, it is tattered and scribbled on, but it is a system that really works for me.

Here is what Martha's planning sheet looks like. She includes the grams of protein in each of her protein foods. Think about how you might adapt this for yourself.

PROTEIN		VEGGIES (GREEN FOOD)
DAIRY, ETC.	BEANS, MISC. STUFF	Broccoli
Egg/6	Tempeh	Cauliflower
Cheese (1 oz)/6	Kidney beans	Onions
Cottage cheese	Black beans	Bell peppers (red,
(½ C)/13	Lentils (1 C)/18	green, orange,
	Protein powder	yellow)
MEATS	(2 T)/25	Tomatoes
Turkey (4 oz)/26	Tofu	Lettuce
Chicken (4 oz)/26		Avocado
Ham (4 oz)/26	NUTS/NUT BUTTERS	Kale, Swiss chard
Pork chop (4 oz)/22	Peanut butter	Celery
Ground Beef	(2 T)/8	Mushrooms
(4 oz)/20	Almonds (⅓ C)/6	Brussels sprouts
Lamb	Almond butter	Asparagus
Boca Burgers		Frozen veggies
FISH		FRUIT
Salmon (3 oz)/23		Bananas
Tuna (4 oz)/26		Apples
Flounder (3 oz)/30		Strawberries
Haddock (3 oz)/16		Oranges
Shrimp (5 large)/16		Lemons
Sole (3 oz)/30		Limes
Swordfish (3 oz)/24		
Trout (3 oz)/20		BEVERAGES
Crab, lobster, clams		Herbal tea
Cod		

WHOLE GRAINS (BROWN FOODS/ HEALTHY CARBS	MISC.	MENU PLANNER

Brown rice
Potatoes
Sweet potatoes
Roots
Whole wheat
   bread
Oatmeal
Quinoa
Wasa crackers
Ry-Vita
Miso
 	
NIGHTTIME CARBS
Potato
Apple
Oatmeal—plain
Triscuits
 	
CONDIMENTS/SAUCES
Salsa
Soy sauce
Olive oil
Canola
   cooking
   spray
	SUPPLEMENTS
	All One Vitamin
	Udo's Oil
	Vitamin C
	B-complex (Twin
	   Labs liquid)
	Salmon oil
	Digestive
	   enzymes
	   (lipase)
	Oat milk
	Soy milk
	Milk
	
	PERSONAL PRODUCTS
	Soap
	Shaving stuff
	Toothpaste
	Hair stuff
	
	HOUSEHOLD PRODUCTS
	Toilet paper
	Kleenex
	Cleaning stuff
		Sunday
		
		Monday
		
		Tuesday
		
		Wednesday
		
		Thursday
		
		Friday
		
		Saturday

Step 4: Take the Recommended Vitamins
and Have a Potato Before Bed

I recommend taking at least vitamins C, B-complex, and zinc. I have chosen these nutrients because they are related to the metabolism of carbohydrates and the synthesis of serotonin from tryptophan. Take 1,000 to 3,000 mg of vitamin C each day, plus vitamin B-complex (choose one that gives you 25 mg of the major B vitamins) and 15 mg of zinc. I like to use a liquid B-complex because you can adjust the dosage more easily if you need to. If you take the zinc as lozenges, you will get an added benefit of enhancing your immunity from inhaled germs that commonly cause colds and flu.

Often clients come into my office with a huge bag full of bottles of vitamins and supplements: "What about taking those supplements that are supposed to reduce cravings, speed metabolism, and all that? Won't those help? Doesn't losing weight require additional things?" I ask them if they have had breakfast with protein that day. Usually the answer is no. So I tell them to focus on the food.

Eat breakfast, have protein with each meal, simplify the vitamins, and let your body heal. Later on, if you wish to add other things, you can do more homework and make informed choices that aren't based on impulse and sugar feelings. But if you are relying on "taking" something to stabilize your body chemistry and help you lose weight, you are going to miss the miracle of using food as your healer.

The Potato

The potato is your evening "pill." You will have a potato with skin on it three hours after your evening meal. You can experiment with the size and type of potato that works for you. The potato serves as serotonin medicine. (It is why my first book is called *Potatoes Not Prozac*.) The protein you have been eating gets tryptophan into your blood. The potato causes a release of insulin to move that tryptophan into your brain to be used by the serotonin factory. This evening carbohydrate is very intentional.

Yes, the potato scores high on the glycemic index and does cause a rise in blood sugar. This is why it is such an effective serotonin medicine. The glycemic index score of carbohydrates has become a buzzword in the last few years. A number of diet book authors have suggested that a food is good or bad based on where it falls on the glycemic index, which is supposed to measure the effect of a given food on the rise of a person's blood sugar after eating that food.

To understand why potatoes have gotten a bad rap, it helps to look at where the glycemic index came from. Before the 1980s, nutritionists working with diabetic patients used to recommend that they eat a certain amount of carbohydrates per day. These were simply defined as different starches and included such things as bread, rice, potatoes, and cereal. They didn't differentiate white foods, or refined, wheat-based foods and simple carbohydrates that trigger a quick rise in blood sugar, from brown foods, or healthy, complex carbohydrates that cause blood sugar to rise more slowly.

In 1981 David Jenkins wanted to test how different starches affected diabetics and to quantify the different impact of the starches on their blood sugar in a comparative index. He published an article in the *American Journal of Clinical Nutrition* and called the index the glycemic index.[23] The glycemic index was designed for diabetics and

was never intended to tell people how to lose weight.
Since that time, a great deal of work has been done to determine the glycemic index score of different foods, so
the index can be a useful guide to identifying foods that
can affect your insulin levels. However, to use the glycemic
index to say, "Don't eat potatoes or carrots, but wine is
okay," as some diets do, seems unrealistic and even coun-
terproductive to healthy eating.

White potatoes *without* the skins score high on the
glycemic index because they do cause a significant rise in
blood sugar. This rise in your blood sugar then causes a
rise in your insulin level. This is exactly what we want—a
timed, intentional rise in insulin. Your body uses this insulin to move the amino acid tryptophan from your blood
into your brain to be used in the serotonin factory. Eating
a potato (*with* skin and some olive oil) on it gives the best
effect—a small rise in blood sugar but not off the scale.
The potato raises your serotonin level without spiking
your beta-endorphin. And the potato will make you feel
comforted and full.

After I published *Potatoes Not Prozac*, a number of people asked me what alternative complex carbs they could
use as their pre-bedtime snack, and so I started to experiment with other foods. Over time I saw that for most people Mr. Spud is hands down the best alternative, but if you
find yourself one night thinking you'll go nuts if you have
to eat one more spud, go ahead and substitute something
else. Eat an apple or 3 or 4 Triscuits; have some oatmeal
or a piece of whole grain toast. And while these are options, remember that Mr. Spud is number one!

If you are diabetic, the rise in blood sugar caused by
the potato will be too intense for you, so you will need to
find another choice. Many diabetics use a sweet potato for

this step, a slice of whole grain toast, or some Triscuits instead. Measure your blood sugar in the morning and see which alternative is best for your body. Pay very close attention so that you do not create a blood sugar crisis.

If you have a problem with arthritis and are sensitive to potatoes (they are part of the nightshade family and may make arthritis worse), then I also recommend you explore some of the alternatives noted above. Some people have found that shifting to a different type of potato eliminates this problem. Listen to your body, be informed, and make a choice that works for you. But if you are simply a sugar sensitive trying to lose weight, stick with spuds.

You may put some tasty things on the potato. I want you to think of it as your natural medicine, but it doesn't have to be *that* medicinal. Use a little olive oil or your favorite salad dressing (make sure it does not contain sugar), some mustard, or some salsa. Just don't use anything that has protein in it: no sour cream, no cottage cheese, no cheese spread.

You do not have to use a huge potato. A medium-size one will do fine. I buy organic baking potatoes because they are smaller—and, I think, tastier—than the huge Idaho russet potatoes the local supermarket carries. Some folks swear by Yukon Golds.

Experiment to find the right size, amount, or kind of potato that works best for you. If you start having wild and woolly dreams, have less potato. If you awaken groggy in the morning, have less. The relationship between the right amount of potato and feeling better in the morning seems to be strong. You should wake up feeling rested and refreshed. You will feel as if your sleep restored you. If you don't, play with the evening spud. The fun part of using the potato is that, unlike other medicines, you *can* play safely with it to find what works for you. You will get pretty quick and surprisingly accurate feedback for your experimentation.

When I first started recommending the potato at night, I assumed that it was a pretty straightforward task. I was wrong on that, and I kept getting potato questions. I finally devoted part of the website to a page called "1001 Potato Questions," and we still add to it. The *Sugar Addict's Total Recovery Program* also includes many of these questions if you want a more in-depth discussion of the use of the spud.

As you work with the first four steps of the program, you may discover that some interesting changes are happening to your body and your life. By having your sweets *with* your meals, you may find you are having fewer. By observing how much white food or refined carbohydrates you eat, you may have already started to make some different choices. Many people find that the next step is actually one of the easiest to do.

Building a Firm Foundation

Now that you have mastered the first four steps of Phase 1 of *Your Last Diet!* let's move on to the next step. Shifting from white foods to brown foods is pretty straightforward.

Step 5: Shift from White Foods to Brown Foods

In this step, you will shift to eating brown things instead of white things. Having browns instead of whites means eating whole grains rather than refined flour products. This may happen all at once, or it may happen over a few weeks. Some of this will depend on whether you live alone or whether you have a family that thinks something other than white bread is very strange.

Sugar-sensitive people are very, very attached to white things. In fact, you may be more attached to white things than to sweet things. You may find it harder to give up wonderful, crusty, rustic Italian bread dipped in olive oil than hot fudge sundaes because your sugar-sensitive body really, really likes that white stuff. But the white stuff acts like sugar in your body. It can trigger cravings and increase your blood sugar levels. This contributes to high levels of insulin that get in the way of your losing weight.

Brown things are less likely to have this effect. Now, brown things may seem more boring. Whole wheat bread doesn't have quite the same kick as warm French bread! But you may discover a remarkable thing when you make the shift. Brown things have a very high comfort effect. Whole grain products are more substantial. It is almost as if your body remembers that this is the way bread should be. Your body may smile rather than resist this shift.

Brown things include: whole grain bread, cereal, pan-cakes, and pasta; brown rice; cornmeal; whole grain tor-tillas (corn or wheat); oatmeal; potatoes *with skin;* sweet potatoes; yams; and beans of all types, including kidney beans, black beans, garbanzos, and lentils. And yes, beans have protein as well as carbohydrate. People who are vegetarian often use beans and rice as a protein source. If you are not a vegetarian using them for your protein, con-sider them a brown thing. Plan on having green, yellow, and red things as well. Mix your vegetables and your brown things to make a nice combination of complex car-bohydrates. A mixture of one-half brown and one-half other colors works well as you get settled into this step.

Some sugar-sensitive people want to fall asleep about thirty minutes after a meal. I call this feeling a "food coma" because there is a particular quality to it—a sense of being overwhelmed by a specific type of sleepiness. It

is as if the brain simply goes into a fog and sleep is the
only option. I first discovered this by accident. I stopped
having wheat and found the food coma disappeared. I
couldn't believe it. Or more aptly, I didn't want to believe
it because I am very attached to wheat. So I kept testing it,
over and over. I smile now to think of this. It is such addictive behavior. But if you have an allergy to wheat, you can
get this effect.

Initially I was cautious in raising this idea with people
when they were starting their food plan because I didn't
want to spook them with the idea of having to give up one
more thing. I have since found that presenting this information simply gives you one more trick for your bag. You
can take a look at it in your journal and decide whether
getting rid of the food coma is worth giving up wheat.
Since there are now all sorts of wheat alternatives available, it doesn't have to be the huge trauma it was five
years ago. When you are ready, you can read the information about food allergy that starts on page 224.

After you have been steady on the first five steps for a
while, you will find that the idea of "having" to give up
sugar has lost its charge. It is remarkable how much of a
non-effect Step 6 becomes when you are steady on the
program. If you are anxious rather than eager about moving to Step 6, don't do it yet. The anxiety means you are
not ready. Step 6 should be simply another adjustment in
the continuum of making change.

Step 6: Stop Using Sugars

You may have rushed right to this step. Right after you
heard about sugar sensitivity, you decided to go for it. You

said, "Let's get rid of that sugar and get moving here!" You are a true sugar-sensitive person: impulsive, all-or-nothing, and wildly enthusiastic.

Don't stop using sugar cold turkey until you have done the preceding five steps because your body will go through drug withdrawal. Follow the sequence, follow the steps, and then go for it. Remember that you have a special body. You respond to things that evoke beta-endorphin more intensely. Sugar evokes beta-endorphin. If you are sugar sensitive, it is likely that you are physically dependent upon sugars because of your response to the beta-endorphin high. Sugar-sensitive people respond to sugars as if they were drugs, and sugar withdrawal can have intense symptoms if you rush into it.

Think of the no-sugar shift as drug detox. Connect this idea of detox to your own body and brain. When you give up sugar, you will be giving up a "drug" that has been very important to you. If you simply go cold turkey without having done the preparation, you are going to be one unhappy pup. You will feel tired, headachy, cranky, and irritable. Your muscles may ache, and you may feel sick to your stomach. You get these symptoms because you have beta-endorphin receptor sites in places other than your brain. When they don't get the "drug" they are used to, they let you know with symptoms.

Going off sugar affects the same biochemistry as going off heroin. Your withdrawal symptoms will certainly not be as severe as those of a heroin addict, but you, too, will be kicking the habit. You may get the shakes, feel nauseated and edgy, or have diarrhea or headaches for a few days. You may be surprised by the intensity of the physical changes you feel. Please, please, please take the detox seriously. Prepare your body and minimize the stress of your detox. Please follow the recommendations I make—they have worked for thousands of people and can work for you.

I *never* thought I could live without sugar. It was my friend, my lover, my comfort. But after I had been doing the plan for a while, I found myself thinking it might be possible. I got braver with each week.

Josie

No Sugar? Ever?

You may fear making the commitment not to have sugar for the rest of your life. In Alcoholics Anonymous people are taught not to think of giving up alcohol for the rest of their lives, but "just for today"—and when things get tough, "just for this hour" or "just for this minute." In *Your Last Diet!* I advocate "one choice at a time." Don't get up each morning thinking, "I won't have any sugar today." Instead, just ask yourself, "What choice will I make this time, this breakfast, this snack?" Remind yourself that no one is asking you never to have sugar again or even to get through the day without some food you need.

Get ready, do your homework, and prepare yourself so that your sugar detox doesn't clobber you. Shift your carbohydrates from white to brown. Eat your sweets at mealtimes. Before you start a sugar detox, you will want to increase your water intake. Drink water every day. Drink eight to ten glasses of water each day (64–80 ounces). If you weigh more than 200 pounds, drink more than that. I use a rough guideline of half your body weight in ounces of water. If you find it hard to drink eight separate glasses of water throughout the day, try filling a 32-ounce water bottle two or three times over the course of the day and simply sip it. Or if you are not a sipper, you may be able to drink little glasses of water. Find the method that works for you, but drink that water. If you have kidney problems or any medical conditions that suggest drinking a lot of water is not for you, check with your doctor as you increase your water.

You may think that you will have to pee all day. But a funny thing happens. As your body gets hydrated, you will be less frantic about peeing. Here are some of the things that water does for you:

- **Carries nutrients to your cells**
- **Carries waste out**
- **Makes chemical reactions work in your brain and body**
- **Serves as a lubricant wherever your body needs moisture**
- **Helps to regulate your body temperature**
- **Fills you up and make you feel less hungry**

Water enhances neurotransmission. Your brain functions with electricity, and water conducts electrical signals. If your brain is dehydrated, the electrical signals won't get transmitted properly. Drink water.

Remember to increase your *water* intake, not just your *fluid* intake. Juices, coffee, milk, tea, and soda do not count as water. In fact, because of the caffeine they contain, coffee, tea, and cola are diuretics—they make your body lose water. In addition to drinking eight to ten glasses of water a day, drink an additional 12 ounces of water for each can of soda or cup of coffee or tea you drink. In other words, subtract the coffee, tea, and cola you drink from your total water intake. Whenever you drink these things, you will have to drink additional water to compensate.

Many people ask me whether it is okay to continue drinking soda. They are used to having soda with their meals, particularly lunch. They ask what to drink instead. I say, "Drink water." They protest, "But Kathleen, water is boring." And I say, "Yup, water is boring." Water is good. Boring water will heal your body. Drink water. You can add lemon if it helps.

Many people have a hard time remembering to drink more water. "I just am not thirsty," they say. It seems that for sugar sensitives, the thirst signal, like the hunger signal, doesn't work the way it should. You don't notice thirst until you are dehydrated or getting a headache. Drink water by the clock rather than by your thirst.

Getting Ready for Your Sugar Detox

When you are ready to start your sugar detox, go back to your food journal. If you don't have a food journal, you aren't ready to do your sugar detox. Go back, go back, you impetuous sugar addict! Do that journal! It's vitally important, especially during sugar detox. If you do have a journal, take a yellow marker and highlight all the sugars you have been using. Include both the foods that you know contain sugars, such as ice cream, cake, cookies, candy, and soda. Then mark the things you think might have sugar but are not sure about. This might include ketchup, relish, chocolate powder for your latte, and salad dressing.

In your detox, you will start by eliminating the known or big sugars. Don't forget that beer and wine are high in sugar. Technically because hard liquor is distilled, it is not a sugar. But the beta-endorphin effect is mighty powerful and will set up huge cravings. The booze has gotta go, along with the candy, cookies, and ice cream. To make the detox successful, you will also want to take all sugars out wherever they are found. The covert sugars hidden in processed food require a little detective work to find them. You will need to read food labels and learn to identify foods where covert sugars are hiding, such as instant breakfasts, tomato soup, bran muffins, protein bars, fruit drinks, and even frozen dinners—places where you never thought sugars would hide. Sugars lurk everywhere.

Food labels can be deceptive. If the chemical structure of a carbohydrate has more than two sugar molecules, it can legally be called a "complex carbohydrate" on a food label instead of a "sugar." So the label may show that a food has no sugar and 35 grams of carbohydrate. But if that carbohydrate is maltodextrin, your body will respond to it as it would a sugar. Watch for words that end in -ose, including sucrose, maltose, and dextrose. They are sugars. Look for words that end in -ol, such as mannitol and sorbitol, because they are sugar alcohols. Things such as concentrated pear juice, date powder, or dehydrated raisin paste are also sugars. Here are a few of the other really sneaky ones:

Date sugar	Maltodextrin
Disaccharides	Microcrystalline
Evaporated cane juice	cellulose
Florida crystals	Monoglycerides
Fructooligosaccharides (FOS)	Monosaccharides
Glycerides	Nectars
Glycerine	Rice syrup solids
High-fructose corn syrup	Sucanat (evaporated
Malted barley	cane juice)

Manufacturers have become very creative in their effort to disguise sugars. Labeling requires that ingredients be listed in descending order of weight. If all the sugar in cereal came from one source, the label would show it as the first ingredient. By using multiple sources, the manufacturer can hide the fact that the first ingredient in a product is really sugar. I once found a protein meal replacement bar with twelve different kinds of sugar. And the label made it sound so healthy! If you don't read food labels, you won't learn the subtleties of where sugars are hidden. If a product is labeled "low fat," the chances are it will be high in sugar.

It is not necessary to be hypervigilant about how much of these covert sugars you still have in your food because your journal will help you know whether they are getting to you. Fewer than 10 grams of sugar may not be an issue, but your body will tell you. If you find yourself getting cranky, feeling edgy, or craving certain foods, and feel that you have been diligent with your program, look for the coverts in places you least expect. Many recovering sugar addicts who talk to each other on the website at www.radiantrecovery.com use oat milk in their morning shake. One of the major manufacturers of oat milk changed the formulation to improve "mouth feel," adding enough covert sugars to raise the sugar content from 12 grams to 19 grams—a 60 percent increase. The sugar-sensitive people thought the new formula was way too sweet, and they noticed it triggered cravings for additional sweet foods. But if they hadn't been paying attention, they might not have figured out that the pretty label change also meant a striking formula change.

How Fast You Go

After you have completed all the preceding steps and are steady on doing the food, you next have to decide how to do your detox. For instance, will you first cut down on sugars and then cut them out completely? Or will you go cold turkey and stop everything all at once? It doesn't really matter which way you go. What matters most is that your detox plan fits what is right for your body and mind.

When I went off sugars I did it all at once, but only after I had done the other steps. However, some people do a detox more gradually and cautiously because it suits their personal style. Baby steps work perfectly for them. While most sugar-sensitive people are impulsive and act like drama pups, there is a subset who are super-careful about making change. They get thrown off balance when too much changes too fast. They take out the biggest sugars before detoxing, and then work on the covert sugars over time.

Which are you? Slow and steady or all at once? Do you want to jump right in, go for it all at once, and then figure out what to do? Or do you want to take those baby steps to get there? Think about how you make other changes in your life. It is important to change your food for detox at this point in a way that works for you. If you use the style that fits your own personality, you will increase the chances that the program will work for you. Your plan needs to fit your style. Later in this chapter I'll help you identify your own style of creating change in your life to help you continue the program after your detox.

Pay special attention to your food during your detox from sugar. Drink lots and lots of water. Fill a liter or quart bottle with water and carry it with you; have two or three whole bottles each day. Drinking water during detox will help you a great deal. You have been doing this already as part of your foundation phase. Increase the amount during detox to help you make the transition more easily. Eat more foods containing soluble fiber, such as apples, oatmeal, beans, and lentils. They will help to maintain your blood sugar and minimize your cravings. Make sure to have regular meals and enough protein at each meal.

> I never thought I could stop eating sugar or white flour because these foods were so connected with feeling good and feeling satisfied. When I was eating them I only noticed the immediate reaction of pleasure and never made the connection to the later feelings of depression, low energy, and irritability. So I started the plan and gradually cut down on sugars and white flours. Eventually I forgot to add sugar to a few items and found I had detoxed for both foods. I felt steady and normal, no big highs and no big lows.
>
> *Suze*

In the first stages after detox, don't think about never having sugar again. That concept is a killer. Don't even consider it. Just let yourself stay focused on one choice at a time. Don't even stretch it to one day at a time. Stick with one choice at a time.

As you walk into the coffee shop in the morning, ask yourself whether you can choose not to have a scone with your coffee. As you are standing in line at the grocery store on your way home from work, ask yourself if you can refrain from buying a Butterfinger to munch in the car.

Don't make the meaning any bigger than each little choice like these or you will scare yourself. If you think about never having sugar again for the rest of your life, you won't go through with this. Going off sugars is a very big deal and you will need to be gentle with the addict in you.

Be careful about the amount of fruit you eat when you are detoxing. Fruits contain sugar, and you are trying to decrease your sugar intake. Don't have any fruit juice at all during your detox because it will trigger your cravings. Later you may decide to add small amounts back in, but for now, stay away from it.

Plan your sugar detox for a time when you are able to manage it without being crazy. The process usually takes five days. The fourth day is often hard. Time it so that on the fourth day you have some space. Do not start your detox so that the fourth day lands on your anniversary or the day you give a big presentation at work. Be strategic. Let your family, friends, and coworkers know what you are doing. Get their support. This is a big step for you. If you do your homework, going off sugar will not be as difficult as you might imagine. And you will feel so much better after you have done it!

Here's how the full sugar detox usually goes:

Day 1: You'll feel excited about getting started.
Day 2: You may begin to feel irritable and edgy.
Day 3: You may be physically uncomfortable, with a headache, joint pain, or an upset stomach. You may feel irritable, angry, tense, or jittery on Day 3. You may have difficulty concentrating or remembering things. You may wonder why you ever started this detox in the first place. Know that this is your sugar-sensitive biochemistry

going through beta-endorphin withdrawal. Know that it
will pass in about forty-eight hours. Hang in there. It's
worth it.

Day 4: This is the hardest day, and it will be crucial to your
detox. If you get really uncomfortable, have *one* piece of
fruit. No, don't eat four bananas. One will do. Remember, you are close to being done.

Day 5: You'll feel great! You'll have energy, and you'll feel
more stable than you can remember. Coming through a
sugar detox will feel good.

Your own detox may take a little more or less time, depending on how much you reduce your sugar intake before you start this last phase. Obviously, if you had already
taken most sweet and white things out of your daily diet
over time, this phase will be pretty simple. If you decided
to be dramatic and go from everything to nothing, you
will have a dramatic detox—you will feel terrible and then
you will feel wonderful. Whatever way you do it, when you
have completed the process, you should feel good. With
sugar recovery, you will need to live your recovery from
sugar sensitivity **one choice at a time**.

If you find that cravings come up after your detox, remember that these happen because something triggered
them. Cravings are a biochemical response to beta-
endorphin priming. They do not simply appear mysteri-
ously out of the blue. Priming happens when a small
amount of the substance wakes up the receptors. They remember how much they liked it, and they start screaming
for more. You are most vulnerable to being primed when
you have been very "clean" for a while. In the early days
after your detox, if you are being very rigorous, you are
most vulnerable to the effects of priming. Those little re-

ceptors remember; they like the drug effect. Give them a little taste and they will have a temper tantrum. You may remember the discussion in the journal section about noticing when you have "just a" little taste of something and then you relapse in a major way. The little slips actually prime you to want more. Paying close attention to what you are eating early on is very important.

If you have a craving, use your journal as a detective tool to uncover what switched it on. Get that ol' yellow highlighter out and work with the journal. You are in charge now. No more learned helplessness in the face of cravings! You are doing a great job. The payoff for getting through a sugar detox is really worth it.

> I felt good yesterday. Good things were happening, but that wasn't it. I just felt like my cells were all happy. I was feeling so good, I was positively radiant! It was affecting people around me.
>
> *Bev*

Finding Your Personal Style of Change

As you work with your journal, you are going to get to know more about your personal style of creating change in your life. This is an important part of the process of getting ready for your diet. You may find that looking at your personal style of making changes in your life is incidental to going on a diet. It may feel like more boring stuff, when you really just want to get on with losing weight. Nevertheless, learning about your style is actually an important piece in succeeding at a diet.

In order for *Your Last Diet!* to work for *you*, you need to adapt it to your own style of doing things, including the way you gather information, the way you learn new things, and the pace at which you handle change successfully. If you understand these components, you will adapt the weight loss part of *Your Last Diet!* in a way that maximizes your success. You are building a repertoire of skills and habits that will truly make this the last time you will *ever* need to diet.

I want to walk you through some ideas I have found really helpful in determining how to create a personalized plan. For instance, the way you gather information and the way you learn things may be very different from the next person's. If you try to use a style that doesn't match your natural way, you will feel uncomfortable. It won't be a good fit. In fact, this is one reason why other diets haven't worked for you. They may seem a whole lot easier than *Your Last Diet!* because you don't have to think and you don't have to plan—you just do what you are told. But if the creators of the diets are telling you to do it in the style that worked for *them*, it is unlikely to be right for you. The content may be helpful, but the way of implementing won't match your needs. In *Your Last Diet!* you are going through these exercises to tease out your own way of doing things. You will then have a clear sense of how to adapt the program to your life.

Gathering Information

People gather information in three ways: through their eyes, their ears, and with their body. You might be a reader, a listener, or a doer. Everyone has a dominant way of gathering new information. People who are readers often have a hard time listening. Listeners have a hard time reading—they love audiotapes and shy away from books. Doers learn from jumping in and doing; the actual experience of using their body to gather information has a huge effect on how much they remember.

Do you know how you best gather information? Spend some time reflecting on it. You may want to write about it. The very best way to gather information is to use all three senses, reading, listening, and doing. When you are gathering information about putting together your own *Your Last Diet!* program, start with your dominant sensory mode and engage the other two to support you.

Here is an example. One of my clients read *Potatoes Not Prozac*. She loved it but had a very hard time remembering what she needed to do. So she got the audiotape version of the book and listened to it while driving. Things started making more sense. Then she went back to the book and highlighted the parts that she liked. She also copied quotes on three-by-five cards that she carried with her. Then she decided to start a support group. She started talking with others about what she had been learning. She used all three of her senses and consolidated the information into a style of changing her moods and her life that worked for her. Using all three modes, her food plan moved from a good idea to a living, working process. She focused on the doing and lived what each of the steps meant to her. And the process finally clicked for her.

Learning New Things

You may not realize that you have many different kinds of intelligence that can help you in making changes. A brilliant psychologist at Harvard, Howard Gardner, has redefined the meaning of "smart" in ways that I find very exciting—and very comforting. Gardner says there are seven different kinds of intelligence. Let me go through them with you.

• The first is linguistic intelligence, or having a way with words. If you have high linguistic intelligence, you like to write and tell stories, you spell well, and you love reading books. I call this **word smart**.

• The second is logical/mathematical intelligence. You are always trying to figure things out. You love computers and mathematical problems and are always asking why. You want to know the reasoning behind any instruction someone gives you. I call this **number smart**.

• The third is spatial intelligence. You are a map lover, a lover of art, slides, movies, and mazes. You draw in your food journal. You loved geometry in high school. You can always tell exactly where the furniture would look best in the living room. You also know how to get the couch through the door even though your husband or wife insists it won't go. I call this **space smart**.

• The fourth is musical intelligence. You have a CD collection, and you may even have your record collection from high school still sitting in the cabinet. You remember all the words to the songs, you sing in the shower, and you play an instrument (although not while singing in the shower). You always have music on while you are cleaning the house. You decide what to play on the car radio. I call this **music smart**.

• The fifth is body or kinesthetic intelligence. You do well in competitive sports. You hike, swim, bike, and in-line skate with abandon. You may fidget and have a hard time sitting still. You like projects such as woodworking, sewing, or carving. You notice other people's movements and gestures. You process information through your body. You get gut feelings about what is the right thing to do. I call this **body smart**.

• The sixth is interpersonal intelligence. You understand people. You know what is going on with everyone. You have an uncanny ability to pick up on someone else's feelings, sometimes even before the other person knows what is happening. You have lots of friends and always seem to be at the middle of a group. I call this **people smart**.

• The seventh is intrapersonal intelligence. You may prefer being alone. You are very connected to your inner world. You are independent and make decisions from a knowing that is very strong for you. You are the ones who march to a different drummer. I call this **creating-your-own-world smart**.

Did more than one of those ring a bell? It should have. We do not have only one type of intelligence. All of us have all seven, but some of these are more developed than others. Let's review them:

- **Word smart**
- **Number smart**
- **Space smart**
- **Music smart**
- **Body smart**
- **People smart**
- **Creating-your-own-world smart**

Let's work with this a bit to see how it can be useful in the process of sorting out your style. Knowing your own strengths will allow you to tap into the parts of you that are the best developed. This is called leading from strength.

> When I looked at my own style, I was surprised by the lack of shame I had in the places where I was weak. I just felt, "This is me, and this is good." It was okay to be strong and weak in different areas and not judge myself harshly.
>
> *Ruth*

At first glance, you may think the idea of being music smart has no relationship to the idea of losing weight. You may be groaning and thinking, "Come on, Kathleen, the diet, get to the diet!" But there is a method to my madness. You know that past diets have not worked. In spite of all your efforts, you are still fat. I am giving you a range of resources that will combine to help you succeed this time, but because this is not a miracle cure, you have to find a solution that works through thoughtful reflection, diligent commitment, and long-term behavior change. This is strategic.

Doing this exercise carefully will help to ground you in your strengths and reinforce your confidence that you have other skills you can draw on to get you through the hard times. This can be as simple as doing something like exercising to music so that you help yourself learn through your music intelligence, or by making graphs in your journal if you learn through numbers. If you are low in body smarts, you can expect that you will feel less competent in that area, so you want to draw from your strength in other categories. Once you have a context in which low body smarts is simply functional and *not* the huge inadequacy that you have always considered it, you will be better able to simply build on the weakness using your strength.

Let me share with you how I used the smarts scale to design my own program. Here's how I rank myself (on a scale of 1–10) on my innate ways of being "smart":

Word smart	10
Number smart	7
Space smart	9
Music smart	1
Body smart	2
People smart	10
Creating-your-own-world smart	10

Now, let's take a look at how I chose these ratings. First, I was always smart in school. That didn't mean I always did particularly well, because if I got bored or I wasn't interested in something, I didn't bother to learn it. But inside, I felt like a smart person because **words** and **numbers**, which is what school is generally about, came easily to me.

I am very **space** smart. This meant that geometry was very easy for me. I sailed through the tenth-grade geometry book in one month. (Let's not even talk about how hard algebra was!). One moving day when I was a young married woman, the big guys with big muscles came to move our furniture out of our second-floor apartment. They got to the couch and were stumped. They must have tried it six different ways. I watched the whole time. Finally I said, "Why don't you just put it up on end and then sort of rotate it through the doorway?" Of course, it immediately fit through, although they didn't want to admit some girl came up with the idea.

On the other hand, until fairly recently I felt really stupid about **music**. I love music, but I could never hear the sound differences that people would talk about. I cannot remember tunes or melodies. I cannot remember lyrics. I even have a hard time with Christmas carols. In fact, as I write this paragraph, I can feel the sadness I have always had about not being music smart.

I have never felt totally comfortable with my **body**. As a youngster, I never played sports and always felt like a klutz. I can remember doing yoga or taking horseback riding lessons and having the instructor say something about feeling a certain muscle in my leg. I would have to really, really work to figure out how to find my leg, let alone adjust a specific muscle. Now, as I work out with weights in the gym, I am a whole lot better with knowing my body. But it was never a natural kinesthetic sense.

I have been **people** smart since I was tiny. My mother told me that even as a two-year-old, I knew what someone was feeling. As a six-year-old, I would walk into a room and tell her how everyone was feeling that day. Of course, she thought this was a little weird, since she was very low in people smarts. People often tell me that they feel understood and heard when they read my writing. Those who are people smart make emotional connections easily.

Most sugar-sensitive folks are people smart. I suspect our lower beta-endorphin makes us more intuitive. Beta-endorphin buffers both physical and emotional pain. Less buffer may well mean more sensitive reactions to feelings. Sometimes they are considered oversensitive. Often sugar-sensitive people turn to sweet or white food to shut down the intensity of the feelings. I consistently hear this from my clients and from people on our forum.

And then we have **creating-your-own-world smart**. I remember my mother scolding me often for being "too independent." She did not create her own world, and my finding my way even as a very little girl made her very uneasy. I marched to a different drummer as soon as I could walk, and I followed what seemed right to me. When I was young, this created enormous problems. In school, I was accused of not following the rules because I ignored the ones I felt were arbitrary and hurtful. In college, I wanted to study philosophy to understand the meaning underlying the way things seem to be. Being independent served me well in graduate school and gave me the strength and focus to create a totally new field, that of addictive nutrition. When one of my advisors said, "You can't name your degree that—no one will know what it means," I replied, "They will in five years." That was creating-your-own-world smart at its best.

Leading from Strength

The most effective way of making change is to lead with your strengths and consciously work to strengthen your weaknesses. Let me give you a concrete example.

After hearing about something called the Mozart effect, which suggested that certain kinds of music can alter how the brain functions, I wanted to learn more about it. Being word smart, I started the process by reading the book *The Mozart Effect*. In doing so, I was leading from strength. Then I got the audiotapes of the book. Then I started listening to Mozart's music while cleaning the house. Now I listen to music on a cassette player while working out at the gym to strengthen my music smarts and my body smarts at the same time! Leading from the strength of my word smarts let me get comfortable enough with the content of the material to push myself into the places where I feel less confident.

Now figure out how you would rate your own smarts, on a scale of 1–10, and fill out the list below. Think about how you know that you have which smarts.

> Word smart
> Number smart
> Space smart
> Music smart
> Body smart
> People smart
> Creating-your-own-world smart

Here is a chart that shows you how a number of people doing the program scored. I found it fascinating to see the different profiles.

WORD	NUMBER	SPACE	MUSIC	BODY	PEOPLE	WORLD
10	7	4	4	2	10	10
10	1	3	10	1	8	2
10	10	10	1	3	10	10
10	1	3	7	2	10	10
6	5	8	6	3	9	10
8	10	10	6	4	9	10
10	0	2	7	10	10	5
5	6	8	10	7	9	5
9	9	7	8	7	6	6
10	10	7	8	7	6	10
10	7	10	6	4	5	8
8	6	1	10	1	7	6
10	7	9	1	2	10	10
10	2	6	4	5	10	10
9	6	9	10	4	10	10

Remember, this is a group of people just like you. Regular sugar-sensitive people with regular lives. People who were overweight and discouraged and who had tried every diet in the world. These are the same people who felt like C57 mice, who felt they had no willpower and were somehow inadequate because they couldn't "just say no." When I asked them to do this exercise and share the results with me, I was struck by the power and grace of what it revealed. The exercise provides perspective about different ways of being in the world. It shows that different is just different—it is not something to be ashamed of. One person noted that the scores helped her to see herself as a mixture of different kinds of intelligence, neither good nor bad, and that looking at herself this way took the sting out of a competitive measure of IQ.

Let me share with you some of the comments these same people made as they did this exercise.

WORD SMART
- I love to read and I spell well, hate to write and can't tell stories well.
- I love writing, talking, debates, dictionaries, good movie dialogue, spelling, poetry, fiction/nonfiction, and communicating with others.
- I write a lot, love to do research, love to think about things and analyze stuff.
- I create stories, and spelling is easy.

NUMBER SMART
- I did real well in math and I ask why a lot.
- I like to know the why of everything, but I have a hard time with (and no love for) math beyond the get-through-life stuff.

- I am a computer programmer and logical but not strong at math-type problems.
- I have researched my family geneaology extensively.

SPACE SMART

- I love old maps, enjoy mazes, and have taken an art class but don't draw in my journal. I love geometry and can tell where the furniture would look best, but I can't get the couch through the door.
- Not much here! I am definitely *not* the one to figure out how to get the couch through the door.
- I loved geometry and I would like to learn how to sculpt, but you would never want me to be the one to tell you where to put the furniture.

MUSIC SMART

- I love music and used to be smart at it when I was young, but I have not cultivated my abilities in many years.
- I am much happier when there is music playing. I almost always have some music on when I am at home.
- I love music and I am very passionate about it.
- On my commute to and from work, or anytime in the car, I sing at the top of my lungs. Believe me, you wouldn't want to be with me—I have no talent. I just love music.
- I need my music—I still have every record I ever bought!
- I used to play the piano, and I still remember the tunes.

BODY SMART

- I am just learning to appreciate how my body can move and how wonderful it is. This is new.
- I love to move and feel deprived when I can't.
- I am very intuitive and get gut feelings. Over the years I have

disconnected from my body. As a young child, I was so in
my body.
- I love to move—to hike, to exercise, swim, play tennis, use
weights, do aerobics.
- I went around for years pretending my body ended at the
first chin!
- I think my body smarts will go up more as I allow my body
expression.

PEOPLE SMART
- I like to have a lot of friends and am at the center of planning.
- This is very strong for me; it is my work.
- This is an important part of my life.
- My people connections provide support and direction to my
finding the best way to be.
- I love being with people, connecting with people, but have to
balance it with time alone to feel grounded.

CREATING-YOUR-OWN-WORLD SMART
- I am very connected to my inner world.
- I make a lot of decisions intuitively and delight in learning
more in this area.
- My alone time is as precious to me as my worldly time.
- I need quiet space like others need sunshine. It is my place of
strength—my power center.
- I don't need to ask others what choices to make. I ask myself
and just "know."

So how do you apply this to your diet plan? It's simple,
though it's going to sound strange at first. If you have
high musical intelligence, for instance, adding music to
your diet is actually going to help you get started. Now,
does this mean you play Mozart while you eat? Or that you

listen to Pink Floyd while you exercise? Possibly, if music smarts are your strongest suit.

Knowing which intelligence is your strong suit can turbocharge the effectiveness of your diet plan. For me, this means charts and graphs *and* people. For you it will mean something else. Lead from your strengths. Get to know them. Rather than staying stuck on feeling inadequate about losing weight, connect with where you shine. Do this exercise and write down what you find. Do not just read it and think it; actually write it out so the data you get really sink in.

• If you have strong **word** smarts, read this book and everything else you can find about sugar and carbohydrate sensitivity. Read *Potatoes Not Prozac* and *The Sugar Addict's Total Recovery Program*. Go to the website at www.radiant recovery.com and read the newsletter. Read the community forum. Let your reading skills enhance your deep mental and physical understanding of the information.

• If you have strong **number** smarts, make charts and graphs as you go. Count things. Get counting software for your computer. Track changes in a quantitative way. Rank your feelings, code your foods. Make lists, keep track. Learn the grams of protein, fat, and carbohydrate you are eating. Use numbers to support your process.

• If you have strong **space** smarts, draw pictures in your journal. Create different spaces for different parts of your program. Use your imagination to form visual images of how you want to be, what you will wear, and how your body will change as you lose weight. Color-code your feelings in your journal. Use highlighters in the book.

• If you have strong **music** smarts, play music while you write in your journal. Play music while you cook. Take music with you while you exercise. Exercise by dancing. Pick the music that makes you feel the best.

• If you have strong **body** smarts, use times when you are moving to learn about the science. Take note cards along to look at while you are walking. Use a new pen for writing the exercises so you are touching words as you read. Write notes in the margins of your books. Read the newsletter from the website while you are walking on the treadmill. Ride your bike while listening to the tapes.

• If you have strong **people** smarts, connect with other people who will support the diet. These may be friends or folks on the www.radiantrecovery.com Community Forum or on one of the online support lists. Start a book study group in your community. Convene a group of friends to do the program with you. Start a food group at your church.

• If you have strong **creating-your-own-world** smarts, create your own special place for your journal, your books, your weight loss "toys" (dumbbells, for instance). Go at your own pace, make your own rhythm. Understand how you are adapting the plan to fit what works for you. Remember to do the plan and not get so creative that you design something that has no resemblance to *Your Last Diet!*

Have fun with the process. Do it when you start out and then do it again over time. Watch how things change as your food changes. Get to know your own personal style and rhythm. Lead from your strengths, and give yourself a boost in the places where you are less developed. Use your best while cultivating your least and you will become ready for the last step—finding radiance. As you connect with who you are from this deeper place, you will discover a kind of continuing smile coming from within. It is subtle and hard to describe, but you will know it as it comes.

4

Getting Steady

When we are in the midst of chaos and the drama of our sugar lives, the idea of steady seems pretty boring. Steady seems pale against the rush of sugar feelings and the desperation of withdrawal. But attachment to drama has changed as you have changed the food in the first six steps of the foundation of *Your Last Diet!* All this preparation has made a difference. The seventh step of getting ready for your diet phase is more about your way of being in the world than it is about your food. It is called finding radiance.

Step 7: Finding Radiance

When you started *Your Last Diet!* you probably felt that if you could lose weight, your life would then work. Many sugar addicts believe this. It is why we quest for the perfect diet, because we think it is the perfect solution. After you have done the first six steps, however, this magical belief

Take Some Time with Your Program

Let your program settle in some. Now, think about where you are in the process of this first part of *Your Last Diet!* Have you been rigorous, detailed, and persistent? Have you dallied, played, or poked around with the steps? Are you still weighing yourself all the time, or are you now being more attentive to how you feel and how your body talks to you? Are you keeping up with your journal? Notice how you criticize or judge yourself. Do you ascribe "good" to rigor and "bad" to dabbling? Listen to your inner judge carefully and discover if she or he is an ally or a saboteur. Is there any difference in how you talk to yourself now compared with when you started the program? I suspect you are kinder to yourself, more understanding and appreciative of your body and its needs.

Work with these inner voices. They are crucial to your long-term success. If the voices are still criticizing you, it is a clue that your food is not yet balanced. But you don't have to push things. Recovery may not work in quite the way you expect. In fact, sometimes diligence is less useful than dalliance. Let me tell you why. For many, many years you have demanded that you be self-disciplined. You have pushed yourself and then felt guilty when you couldn't do what you demanded of yourself. Yet I hope that *Your Last Diet!* is showing you a different way of working with yourself, your body, and your food. You have already improved your relationship to your body and your way of making changes in your life. You have thrown out or modified your old idea of what a diet is or has to be. You have taken your time in coming to terms with each step. You have been mindful and have let your own knowing guide you in your readiness for moving to the next step. You have been a different kind of diligent and learned to listen to what your body is teaching you about its needs. To others, this may appear to be dalliance—but the improvement in your mood and energy prove it's not!

When I first started doing my own plan, I thought that getting the program meant doing it fully, following the instructions, and not poking around. I still held the belief that being disciplined and rigorous was the only way to go. Now I see that *Your Last Diet!* works when that something else is operating, something a little more subtle and unexpected. Just showing up and being in relationship to your body will help you more than being tough on yourself. Here's how I got to thinking this way.

I used to lead a ten-week guided imagery course called "Finding Healing from Within." Each week we would do a guided meditation. After the meditation, the participants would draw what they had experienced, seen, or imagined, and the group would share their feelings. Some group members would sleep through every single meditation and make up a drawing because they had no memory of anything in the meditation. This made me really uncomfortable. Was I failing these people? Were they failing the group? Were they in denial? How could they sleep through my wonderful imagery?

At the end of ten weeks we reviewed the progress of everyone in the group. How had they changed? How did they feel? Surprisingly, time and time again, the sleepers would have as remarkable a change in feelings as the doers. Not once, not twice, but every single time. Ten weeks of sleeping through and they would report a profound sense of inner healing. They didn't "work it." They slept through the meditations on a conscious level. But they were there. They showed up and they drew the pictures and they talked about what they had experienced.

The sleepers taught me something. The simple act of showing up, of being present, creates change. It creates powerful change even if on the outside it may not seem so. Making a commitment to healing starts a process—a chain of events that is much deeper than we may think. When you say, "I will get better," when you begin to hold the idea of "I will do whatever it takes," something inside you starts to shift.

Once I realized this, I had to reexamine how I approached and followed the seven steps of healing sugar sensitivity. What was happening when I was playing around? Could those times be like the sleeping times in my guided imagery class? Could change be happening in spite of what seemed to be inattention? I looked in my journal and discovered something astounding. When I was writing in my journal, attending to the steps, listening to my body, even if I wasn't doing it perfectly, change was happening. I was making progress even when I was being kinda sloppy.

Think of the sleepers who were there in the room with the group practicing guided imagery. Every week they woke up, colored with the group, and talked about sleeping. When I showed up, kept the journal to listen to my body, and wrote about sleeping through my food plan, I was still engaging with my body and working the steps. I was talking with myself about what was happening. I was not criticizing myself for "food sleeping"; I was simply watching. And I kept coming back to the journal. I kept coming back to my body and my healing.

The nature of the unhealed sugar-sensitive person is to give up when things or feelings get difficult. Like the

C57 mice, we used to crouch in the corner and think we couldn't stick to a plan. Our unhealed biochemistry reinforced our feelings of inadequacy, being overwhelmed, and inability to follow through. A thousand failed diets from the past strengthened these feelings even more. As soon as we "sleep," or fall off the plan, we say, "See, you did it again!" We dropped whatever food program we were on and ran away from ourselves.

However, now that you are on *Your Last Diet!* you know that you can keep going. You know how to face your resistance, talk to your inner voices, go slowly, do the food, and listen to your body. Knowing you are sugar sensitive lets you finally understand what to expect from food. Here you are, healing yourself, feeling better, staying the course. Think of that. You are actually tenacious. You may be impulsive and impatient, but you can be and are committed to finding a solution.

Your Last Diet! helps you use your tenacity in a new way. You are settling into a routine that will support your weight loss and an entirely new way of being in the world. Because you now finally understand why other diets haven't worked, you can start to make choices. You can change "I know this won't really work" into "Hmmm, let's sort this out. Why am I bored? Why don't I like the journal? Why do I sabotage my efforts?" Asking these questions becomes a part of your healing. You are questioning, not listening to the old voices of inadequacy. Sorting them out patiently before moving on to the weight loss part is *not* dalliance. It is commitment.

To deepen your commitment in the last stages of your preparation for Phase 2 of *Your Last Diet!* say to yourself, "I will do whatever it takes to heal my sugar sensitivity. I will give it time, money, energy, whatever it takes. Taking care of my food will be at the top of my list. Not after my job, or after my family, or maybe when I get to it. But every day." This affirmation is different from others. Generally, when you make affirmations, you make them in your head—you think about them. But what does it really mean to do whatever it takes?

Doing what it takes means something different for everyone. Let me share what it means for me. It means I still write in a food journal. Even though I know what I eat and I know what it means, I do it. And I read my journal and study it. It means looking in my refrigerator and planning my food. Do I have the stuff for lunch tomorrow? Do I need to make an extra portion at dinner to have at lunch? Do I need to go to the grocery store? How and where will I cook tomorrow? Which restaurant are we going to? Will they have food choices for me? Former worries about my inability to manage my food and moods have shifted into reflections on what I *can* do every day: what I will eat, when I will eat, where I will eat.

I now think less and do more to make my food plan work. Every day, any moment one of those "I just can't do it" thoughts creeps in, I replace it with an action thought. I do whatever it takes to stay steady on the steps. I just do the food. And the miracle of my own healing continues— my energy doesn't fade, my humor flows, my temper is even, my moods and focus stay steady, and I stay connected to my true self.

Ask yourself what you need to do to act on this affirmation. In which of the six steps you've done so far do you need to go slower? In which do you need to be more rigorous? Are you forgetting to eat breakfast on time? Are you leaving breakfast "just a" little later while you take care of other things? Are you skimping on the amount of protein you have for breakfast? Do you need to shop for enough oatmeal, eggs, or sausage on the weekends? Are you up-to-date with your supply of morning protein shake? What do you need to do to tidy up breakfast?

Is your journal a joyful part of your daily routine? Do you do it every day? Are you not only writing in it but using it to understand patterns? Can you see the changes you have made? Are you excited about your growth? Are you compassionate about your slips? Do you get right back on track? Can you recognize danger times before they create problems?

Are you eating meals at regular times? Are the intervals short enough to keep you from slipping? Are you having to juggle your schedule, or do you have a solid routine every day? Do you plan for the unexpected—having to work late, having a soccer game run over? Do you make sure that meals, good meals, are on time and meet your needs?

Are you regular with your vitamins and your potato? Have you found the size and type of potato that works perfectly for you? Do white things slip in at unexpected times, or do you remember to pay attention? Do you have backup plans for potlucks, parties, and family gatherings? Have you developed effective responses to the folks who want to derail your program?

Take time to really reflect on how you are changing. The foundation work is a time for the joy that comes with healing your sugar-sensitive biochemistry. Mary once described herself as a fat C57 mouse sitting on a very wobbly three-legged stool trying to keep her balance. As she did her program, her image changed. The mouse was still fat and still sitting, but the stool was steady and the mouse was squeaking out a wonderful song. Find your own images to celebrate what is happening. It is very powerful and very special. Mark this time.

Going Back to Your Body in a Loving Way

When you got started on *Your Last Diet!* you, like me, no doubt had lots of self-hate and frustration about your body. Much of that was colored by your sugar feelings. Now that those are quieted, I want to take you back to your body and have you reconnect with it from this steady place.

All the understanding and good food in the world will not help you feel better and lose weight in the long term if you are not truly in relationship to your body. Your journal has given you a way to look at your eating patterns and the connections between what and when you eat and how you feel. Now we want to take this listening one step deeper. Being in a relationship with your body is the same as being in a relationship with another person. You spend time with the other person, listen to what she or he has to say, and pay attention to his or her needs. You are going to learn to do all these things with your body.

Your body believes that its most important job is to take care of you. Yes, even your fat body, the one you have such a hard time with, cares about you. That body has your best interests at heart. I understand that this is a very radical concept to you because you are used to feeling disgust, repulsion, or frustration when you look at your body. It may be inconceivable that the very body with which you have struggled so much and that you have avoided so diligently might have something helpful to offer you.

Listen to Your Body

Your body wants to talk to you. But as we saw earlier, your body does not talk in words. It talks in symptoms. Sometimes it talks with a subtlety that you will miss if you are not paying attention. So your next task is to learn the language of your body on a deeper level. You do this through your food journal. Your food journal is your most powerful ally in being able to lose weight successfully.

You may have kept other journals in the past. Many diet plans ask you to record what you are eating, but often you just calculate calories or fat grams. That kind of journal can be boring and nonproductive. Counting is not a relationship. Counting distances you from your body and from listening to your body.

The journal you have started in *Your Last Diet!* is a sort of code book. Your body's symptoms and feelings are a code, a unique language. Because your body doesn't "talk" in English, Swedish, Spanish, or whatever language *you* speak, you are going to have to learn its vocabulary. You will become a code breaker by listening, recording, and experimenting.

Denial Keeps You Safe

Often when people get to this stage of the plan, they do very well at recording their meals and feelings, but they don't have as much skill at interpreting their notes when they read over them. For instance, you may have kept a record of what you eat and how you feel in your journal, but you may not have wanted to look at it or review it a whole lot. This may reflect denial about really wanting to know your feelings. This is a very common realization to run into at this stage, just as it was in the second step when you began keeping your journal.

Don't beat yourself up. Your emotional relationship to food, to eating, and to your body has been highly charged for many years. The feelings may be painful. Listen to your resistance. It is a gift. It is telling you how many feelings are wrapped up in food and your body. On some level, you know that if you look closely at your food, you might have to change even more. The idea of more change may scare you, but remember you want to do whatever it takes. Make one choice at a time and go slowly. Work according to *your* style of making change.

Not looking, or denial, is what has kept you safe from the feelings of pain, shame, and rage that you carry about your weight. Denial is not a horrible thing. Denial is what allows you to function when things feel out of control. If you feel hopeless and overwhelmed, if you feel that nothing is going to work for you, then denial allows you to function. If you don't look at what upsets you, you can manage. If you don't look in the plate-glass window, if you don't look at what you are eating, you are able to get by.

Denial is seductive, persistent, stubborn, and very, very clever. You first met your denial in Step 2 when you started your journal. Perhaps you started working with it then, questioning it, asking this part of yourself what it needs. In this way, you don't get rid of denial so much as redirect its energy. Instead of expending a huge effort to avoid looking at your food or food journal, you take this effort and devote it to serving your healing.

It is critically important to form a relationship with the part of you that has been in denial, the one who has protected you for all these years. The one who has protected you from the feelings of hopelessness and despair about being overweight or out of control around food is going to have a lot to say. And you need to have a way to listen. You want to learn the code so you can understand what your body is saying.

Food has been a comfort. It may have been the one true friend, lover, and companion of your life. It has given you confidence and raised your self-esteem. It has helped you handle stress, quiet your fears, and ease your inner turmoil. Food is a very big deal. People who are neither fat nor sugar sensitive do not understand this. They think weight is a much simpler issue than it is. They don't have a clue.

Being in relationship with your body and honoring food's power in your life will help you stay steady and heal. If you try to lose weight *without* making this connection to the part of you that needs the companionship and support that food has given, it will rebel and tell you in no uncertain terms that it will not cooperate with you on this next phase of your plan. It will get scared that things are going to be taken away, and it will sabotage your plans in a flash.

The Gift of Resistance

If you forget to review your journal or never quite get to that task, it may not be because of denial so much as its close cousin, resistance. You may resist wanting to hear your body's voice because you don't want to hear what it has to say. You avoid the dialogue by not using your journal in this way. What if you were to think of your resistance to using your journal as a gift instead? The fact that you are not doing something doesn't mean you are inadequate. It means that something in you resists the action.

If you can take away the negative spin you have about resistance, you can find a helpful store of energy. Resistance can mark something that is charged, something that is important to you. Bigger resistance means bigger importance. If you are *not* doing something such as using your journal to get to know your body, particularly if you are not doing it while you are affirming you want to, this points out a good lesson. Your mind says you should use your journal more, but you don't. Instead of beating yourself up, bless your resistance as a way to discover something that has a lot of energy for you. The energy locked up in your resistance is important. It can bring you valuable insight. It can teach you something that nothing else can.

In order to get insight about your own resistance, look at it in a new light. Start with allowing the possibility that it has something to offer. Think of your resistance as a very kind, loving, powerful part of yourself. Somewhere along the way, this part got the idea that keeping you safe and comfortable is a very important job.

If you are in withdrawal and are cranky and irritable, this part knows that having something sweet or having some bread would make you feel better. It wants you to feel better. But here's the problem: **Resistance doesn't know.**

The part of you that is resistant doesn't know about sugar sensitivity. It only wants you to feel better and knows that if you drink soda, you'll feel better. It works on very concrete, specific information. It believes its logic is right. It doesn't want you to suffer with crankiness or foggy thinking. The resistant part has your well-being at heart, and it is one smart, creative, tenacious puppy. Your resistance will cut deals, make you forgetful, distract you, cajole you—in short, it will do anything to subvert your changing the rules.

The most effective tool your resistance has is its cousin, denial, which says, "Just one cookie won't matter." Denial says, "You don't really need to use that journal. You know what you eat. You have done this a hundred times. You are a pro. Just avoid sugar and you will be fine." Denial, too, is seductive, persistent, stubborn, and clever. It runs in the family.

Now that you have a new way of seeing resistance and denial as your allies, you can get to know them better and more intentionally. Use your journal to see where and how they work in your life. As your brain and body become less foggy, you can learn more about where and how your resistance works. Martha, who has been on *Your Last Diet!* for two years, once said, "It isn't in the pages where I am diligent so much as the pages where I am sloppy that I see how I get into trouble. I start having some white things, one scone, and I 'forget' the rest of the day."

Look for patterns. You may think it is stress or hard feelings that make you forget. Your journal will show you that your food gets wobbly first and *then* you forget. The wobble always comes first. If you are looking for denial and resistance in your journal, look for wobbly food. Denial and resistance always follow.

Humor these protective energies. They are the markers of when you are in trouble. Invite resistance and denial to dialogue with you. Act as if they were real people with a voice. Ask them what they fear. Negotiate a truce and then get them on your side. Find out what is underneath their fear and address those concerns. Let them know you are not going to allow them to run your life anymore. Just be clear about the fact that yes, you are going to move to the next step (that part is not negotiable) and

you really want to use the energy you used to put into resistance and denial to help you move forward.

For instance, for many months I did not want to write
my feelings in my journal because I didn't want to see how
angry I was about being sugar sensitive. I was enraged that
I had this so-called special body and that I couldn't be like
everyone else. If I opened the door to the feelings, the
rage came spilling out. But at the time I didn't understand why I had such a hard time with the journal. I
thought I was simply forgetting to write. Then I thought I
was resisting. I finally figured out that I was resisting because I didn't like what came up. Once I understood this,
I did some work on my fear of being that angry. All of a
sudden I could journal just fine.

Remember, resistance is a gift.

Nothing Is Lost

None of the effort you have made is wasted. Not one diet,
not one book, not one support group, not one regained
pound has been without a purpose in your healing. Each
effort has given you something. Each experience has
added a piece to understanding yourself and your body.

We have discussed the down side of sugar sensitivity's
biochemistry, so let's spend some time on the up side. I
now have thousands of stories from people who have
healed their sugar sensitivity. The more than 100,000 letters posted to the www.radiantrecovery.com community
website have convinced me that most sugar-sensitive people are smart and creative. Our conversations have taught
me how understanding our unique biochemistry also
gives us a way to make sense of all that past groping for an

answer through multiple diets. It allows us to understand why the Atkins plan worked for a while, or why we slipped, or why we regained weight, or why we were moody even though we were thin.

Yet the work you are now doing is transformational beyond anything you imagined a diet or food plan could offer. Taking this time to get steady does not just ensure that the weight loss phase will work. It is also designed to give you a chance to practice living this new way of being in the world. It's designed to get you radiant and keep you that way!

When I say that nothing is lost, I mean it. As your biochemistry changes, a kind of tolerance and loving will emerge. New feelings will be directed at yourself, your past. Let me give you an example of how this works. A few years ago I spent several months putting together some photo albums. I think it was one of those midlife things we do. When I found some pictures of my fat self, I wanted to croak. Or at least I wanted to rip them up. They reminded me of all the pain and the shame of that time. But I told myself I needed to put them in the album. I realized that even though I wasn't happy about how I looked and I had a hard time remembering the shame, it was still a part of who I am.

As I was finishing *Your Last Diet!* my publisher asked about a set of before-and-after pictures. I acted cool in my first response and then went into a panic at the idea of revealing my "before" self. But I went back to the album. I got one of the the offending pictures out. I figured I was desensitizing myself. I decided to take the picture to the seminar Radiant Recovery does at Ghost Ranch every year. Then I decided to do something really outrageous. I took the picture of my fat self to the copy center and asked them to blow it up to a three-foot-by-two-foot poster.

When we all talked about the picture at Ghost Ranch, people pointed out something I had never seen. I wasn't the only one in the picture. My three kids were there. And there is so much love in that picture, it floors me. I never saw the love; I only saw the shame. Now I see myself as fat but in the midst of love and joy. So instead of losing that time, instead of ripping up the image, I can go back to it and claim the rest of what was there. This is what I mean when I say nothing is lost.

As you get ready to shift into losing-weight mode, you will draw from the experience and efforts you have made for many years. All the failures will provide instruction on what can work for you. Being steady will give you a way to feel empowered and diligent. Having a solid foundation means you can sort out what works for you and actually do it.

Your personal sugar-sensitive weight loss story may be quick and effortless or very slow and arduous. You may have seen dramatic weight loss even as you have been working the seven steps. Or you may need to work really diligently at your weight loss and get steady results over a long period of time. Some people just do the seven steps for stability and lose weight right away. Their weight loss follows effortlessly. Others have to work on losing weight for a very long time. Your genes, your sex, your hormones, your dieting history, your emotional history, and your degree of sugar sensitivity all affect the amount of effort it takes to lose weight.

Losing weight successfully will ask—no, it will *demand*—that you understand and work with each of these factors. Losing weight requires attending to way more than just the food. Each of the variables is like a dot in a big grid. Your job will be to connect the dots. Being steady will give you the capacity to do this.

You may find that you want to or have to explore every single piece of the weight loss plan to get the results you want. This can be really hard work and takes a huge amount of commitment. You need to have the willingness to do whatever it takes. If you haven't changed your bio-chemistry to create the ability to stick with it, no diet plan in the world will work.

But if you have done the seven steps—the foundation food plan—and have been steady for a couple of months, you will be able to stick with what it takes to lose weight. That is the part that is so extraordinary about this plan. It gives you the ability to hang in there. It gives you the ability to stick with the program in a way that would have been inconceivable on any other diet. The miracle that comes with *Your Last Diet!* is not the food in the diet per se; it is the total package that gives you the ability to make the changes. There is nothing magical about the food part of *Your Last Diet!* It is simply a refinement of what you are already doing. The magic comes in the total package. And you are starting to understand this.

You Shift Your Thinking About What Is Important

You used to feel that you didn't have the discipline for diets. You thought you were impulsive and couldn't stick it out. You thought you were impatient and not able to focus. You thought that the problem was you. Well, the problem *was* you, but not in the way you thought. By having done Phase 1 of the plan, you have shifted your body chemistry, your behaviors, and how you view yourself. You have become a radiant, funny, tenacious being—still tubby perhaps, but feeling good about who you are. And this radiant, tubby person says, "Hey. Wait a minute. I want to be who I am. I want to lose weight so I can *move.* I want to lose weight so I can be healthier. I want to in-line skate and swim and dance. I want to hike and keep up with my kids or my grandkids. I want to make love and be goofy. I want to travel, to fit in the coach seats, to ride my bike in Europe."

This is not the same as saying, "If only I could lose weight, I would feel okay about myself." This is "I feel great about myself and I want *more!*"

Change the Food and Change Your Life

How can I explain the power of this shift to you? When it happened to me, I thought it was just me. When it happened with my clients, I thought it was my clinical skills. I finally figured out it is the food! Change the food and you change your feelings about yourself, your body, and what you care about. **Change the food and change your life.**

You may ask me when you should start the weight loss phase. You are ready to lose weight when it no longer matters to you in the same way. When you have shifted from desperation and despair into clarity and motivation. When you have shifted from addiction to recovery. When you are ready to make the commitment to do whatever it takes. When doing the food is a way of life, when it is effortless and skillful. When you want your body to fit who you are inside.

Once you are ready, you will need to accept that you won't know how the process will unfold until you do it. I cannot guarantee that you will lose thirty pounds in thirty days, and in fact, I surely hope you won't! How your body has responded to the foundation work will give you some clues for how you will lose weight. For instance, you may have lost weight when you stopped grazing or bingeing, or when you took out the sugars. Or you may have even gained a little. Or you may have been losing slowly and steadily. Your early response will give you some clues, but it won't tell you the whole story. The weight loss part is different from what you have been doing. And the styles of the people doing *Your Last Diet!* differ tremendously.

I have seen a number of patterns as I have worked with folks over the last fifteen years.

• The **easy players**. They do the basic stability food plan with no trouble; they get clear and focused right off the bat. They don't do the exercises and don't think the emotional part has much to do with them. They lose weight without looking back and think the plan is a good diet.

• The **steady workers**. They do the basic stability plan without a whole lot of difficulty. They get steady and clear but don't really lose weight. They start exercising regularly. They begin to lose weight without a whole lot of effort. They feel better and better each month and find that the combination of the new way of eating and daily exercise is enjoyable and fun. The combination works for them.

• **The scared ones**. They start the basic stability plan and they struggle. They are eating three times a day, as directed, but are still using sugars and white flour products.

They actually gain weight in the first week or two, freak out, and feel out of control and hopeless. They make no connection with others in the process. They continue to feel isolated and angry. They give up on the plan and decide it doesn't work.

• The **committed ones**. They start off not knowing if the plan will work for them. They are not particularly enthusiastic. But they believe in the idea and the science. They do what they are supposed to, and it doesn't work the way they had hoped, but they stick with it. They recognize that their bodies were abused for many, many years. A thousand diets, unhealthy, excessive, pushing it to the max or doing nothing for years changed their body chemistry in a big way. But they keep at it, one variable at a time. Diligently doing detective work, they build an understanding of why this body doesn't budge. They just keep chipping away at what needs to be done. They aren't exactly joyful, but they get results.

• The **willing ones**. They know immediately that the book was written for them. They are enthusiastic and excited. They start the basic stability plan, struggle, and gain some weight in the beginning. They get scared, but they talk to other people on the plan, listen and learn, and hang in there. They learn to use the journal. They start to understand what happened. They get stubborn and stick with it. They get support to get them through the hard part. They ask questions. They learn about their body and they get stable. They make the adjustments and are willing to learn as they go. Their enthusiasm grows and nurtures their diligence. They too get the results they want.

• The **radiant ones**. These are the folks who do the food, make a commitment, and learn to be willing and take the program deeper. They understand that weight loss is one tiny variable in what the plan offers. They embrace the ideas, live them, share them, and shine.

But let's go now to exploring your weight loss. You are ready and you are mobilized. You may find that you have a piece of some of each of these weight loss personalities, or that your style changes as you do the food. Enjoy getting to know how you function and how it affects your behavior.

Shifting into Diet Mode

The very things that have made you crazy can make you whole. You now can see that when you change what and when you eat, you change your sugar-sensitive biochemistry, and your life starts to change, too. You do not have to spend years trying to unravel all the whys of being fat.

The very same body that had an addictive relationship to food is now guiding you into healing. Your addictive personality was willing to go to any lengths to get you what you needed to make you feel better. You simply needed to give it a new job description: healing rather than addiction. The experience you have in changing the food and holding it steady will now serve you in losing weight. Your skill at doing the food is the foundation for your weight loss.

By doing the food and setting the foundation, your sugar-fed impulsivity has quieted so that you can lose weight gradually. "Right now" and "all at once" will not work for weight loss. The ability to go slow and stay steady will serve you well. In this chapter, you will be getting ready for your diet by figuring out what makes it hard for you. You'll be doing some more thinking and writing, but with a different focus.

Get yourself a new notebook that you like. This will be your diet workbook. Committing to weight loss may bring up some feelings that you need to heal, and you are going to work with them in this new notebook. You have carried a lot of baggage, both literally and figuratively, for a long time. The feelings that come up when you try to take the weight off may be intense and scary. You may have been using your eating and your weight to keep yourself away from painful feelings. If your weight loss is to be success-ful, you will need to heal these feelings as part of your plan.

I am not suggesting that you need years of therapy or that you have to digress and get all the feelings fixed be-fore you can lose weight. But I am saying that acknowledg-ing the feelings and working with them are critical parts of the total weight loss picture. I have developed a set of exercises to help you do this. The exercises are simple, straightforward, and not scary. Some of them may be un-comfortable or seem a little weird at first, but everyone who has done them, including many of the online mem-bers of the *Your Last Diet!* program, report that they are exciting and productive. They make a difference.

These exercises will help you create a weight loss solu-tion that works specifically for you. Remember that *Your Last Diet!* is not a magic diet. It is a plan to keep you in a healthy relationship with your body and your food.

The first step toward healing the shame of being fat is to desensitize yourself about your weight. Speak your truth; start by naming things as they are. This simple act can start taking off the huge negative charge you have about being overweight. For example, I prefer the phrase "really, really fat" to "morbidly obese." I hated being "husky" in grade school—being "fat" would have felt cleaner. Remember that here, in this plan, you are among friends. At a recent Ghost Ranch seminar for Radiant Recovery community members, we had fifty people sitting in a room getting to know one another. Someone commented that she liked being in a place where she didn't have to worry about sucking in her stomach all the time. We all laughed at the truth of that.

Let's just call ourselves what we are. Using the word "fat" as we start to talk about weight loss can be a little uncomfortable at first, but it will grow on you. And you may discover that it comes as a great relief.

If you are *very* overweight, this idea of naming the truth may be extremely hard for you. When we set up a special email list on the website for people who were more than a hundred pounds overweight, one of the participants really argued with me about naming it "bigones." She didn't like that name at all. Not at all. Over time, however, it started to feel friendly and comforting to her. The term is a functional description of being bigger than many of the other people in the community, and using it helped to take the negative spin off the reality she had wanted to deny for such a long time.

If you are not particularly overweight but are filled with shame and ambivalence about your body, speaking the truth about what you see will also help. One of our members, who carried about fifteen extra pounds, hated, hated how her stomach was. She felt that because she had skinny legs and arms, everyone noticed this pouchy stomach. She felt she couldn't complain about this because she wasn't as fat as many of the others in the program, but her pain was just as real for her. As she was able to share her feelings and speak what was true for her, she was able to be clear about what she wanted to do.

The next tasks will help you sort out what is right for you. We are going to start with some data collection—getting the facts. Then we will look at some of the feelings. While we are doing this, *keep doing the food.* Hold things steady while you learn more about yourself.

Your Diet Workbook

Get out your diet workbook. Do not use your food journal. Your workbook will hold the writing exercises you are going to learn to do below. It will also record the details of your progress as you shift into diet mode. Make sure you do each entry, but do not try to do them all at once. You may even spend several days on each entry. Take time to really reflect on each one. You do not even have to do them in order, and you can skip around if you like—unlike doing the seven steps of Phase 1! You may want to use a notebook that will allow you to rearrange the material as you work on it, such as a three-ring binder that allows you to move the pages around. You may find that different sections of these exercises affect you more deeply. *Continue to keep your food journal as you work with the diet workbook.*

Entry #1

Write **why you want to do this plan**. Start with what you think will change as you lose weight. Go into detail. Be specific. If you will be able to fit into the special clothes sitting in the back of the closet, write about it. If you will be able to get a husband or wife, or boyfriend or girl-friend, write about that and how it makes you feel. If you will be able to fit in the coach seats of an airplane, write about it. Do pages and pages and pages. Let yourself explore all the beliefs you have about what will change when you lose weight. Imagine losing not just a few pounds, but getting to your ideal weight. Identify the health benefits, the feeling benefits, and the practical benefits. List all the things you have not allowed yourself to dream.

Entry #2

Tell the **story of your weight** from your earliest memories to the present. Include every diet you have ever tried, the total number of pounds you have lost and gained, and where you are now. Go back to the earliest diet you can think of—maybe that grapefruit and cottage cheese diet in the sixth grade. Write down which diet worked for a while, how much weight you lost, and then how long it was before you gained it back.

Draw a weight time line. Start with the earliest diet and then work your way forward. Put the year and the plan. Here is a sample:

1961: Cottage cheese and grapefruit diet
1965: Crash starvation diet before wedding
1970: Supervised low-fat plan
1978: Tarnower's *The Scarsdale Diet*
1979–1985: Assortment of fad diets
1990: Overeaters Anonymous
1991: Weight Watchers
1991: The Hellers' *The Carbohydrate Addict's Diet*

1992: Atkins' *Dr. Atkins' Diet Revolution*
1993: Ornish's *Eat More, Weigh Less*
1994: Phen-fen
1995: Sears' *The Zone*
1996: The Eadeses' Protein Power
1997: D'Adamo's *Eat Right 4 Your Type*
1998: DesMaisons' *Potatoes Not Prozac*
2000: DesMaisons' *The Sugar Addict's Total Recovery Program*

Keep at this; you will remember new diets as you work with your time line. Include all the plans you have tried: Jenny Craig, hospital plans, fat farms, spas, Overeaters Anonymous. Identify the books you have read: Spillman, Pritikin, Ornish, Atkins, Sears, the Hellers, the Eadeses, Sommers, the Chub Club, all of them. If you don't remember and have gotten rid of the ones that were in your personal library, go to the city library and look them up, check them out on your computer, or go to an Internet bookstore and do a search on diet books.

Include how much weight you lost with each plan. Total up the total number of pounds you have lost in your lifetime. Include your current height and weight. Write down how you feel as you review this part of your life's journey. If you start to beat yourself up, stop. This exercise is not a measure of your success or failure. It is designed to help you connect with the diet expertise you have accumulated. When you were doing these diets, you didn't know what you know now. You didn't know you were sugar sensitive. You thought it was your fault, but it wasn't. You simply didn't know. Now you do. And you will have all that skill and expertise in dieting at your disposal to help to shape the personal plan that will work for you.

Entry #3

In Chapter 3, you spent a good deal of time thinking about your style of making changes. Let's revisit that information now with an eye toward getting ready for weight loss. Write about your life and the social and individual factors that will help support the diet phase of your program. Include influences such as job stress, support from your family (or lack of it), money, space, time, and so on. How are you going to draw from your strengths to help support your weight loss? Which of your intelligences will help to anchor you?

Because so many sugar sensitives have strong interpersonal intelligence, you may discover that having personal support is crucial for your success in the next steps. Many *Your Last Diet!* members have organized in their local areas to meet face-to-face. They started with an online group such as Radiant New England or Radiant San Francisco Bay Area and talked with one another through email. They planned potlucks and hobby days and then regular meetings to discuss the books. There were no groups in Idaho, so one woman started a book study group and advertised in her local paper. She wanted real, live people and found them.

Spend some time on this one and think about which of these is most helpful to you.

Entry #4

Write about a change that you have made in your life that was hugely successful. Remember something that worked really well, such as a job, a hobby, a club or group, a move, a creative endeavor, or a volunteer event for your church. Examine the situation and identify the factors that made it work. What were the concrete, specific things you did to create that success?

When I was getting ready to build a website, I knew nothing about Web-based business. I started by simply looking for sites that I liked. First I identified the styles I liked. Then I picked the five I liked the most. Then I sat down and identified the specific things that I liked about each and narrowed my list to four or five things that were really important to me. Then I thought through the financial issues and other logistics that would affect my ability to create the style and function that I wanted. I had a clear picture of what the end product would feel like, although I wasn't sure how to get there. So I moved from a sense of it to a clear design that allowed me to find the right people to make it happen.

When I did this exercise, it helped me see how intentional I have been with those things that worked for me. Martha, who showed us her shopping list in Chapter 2, went through a similar process in looking for a way to plan her food. She started by writing things in her regular calendar, but it got too messy. She listened to someone talk about his shopping list, and she incorporated that into her plan. She made up a system that worked on paper, tried it out, and refined it. After she bought a little hand-held computer, she adapted the plan to fit it. Now it is a part of her daily life.

Shift gears and pick a change you made in your life that did not work at all. Write about how this unsuccessful attempt was different from the successful change. What got in the way of your success? Time? Energy? Other commitments? Put it all down.

For instance, I had dreams of making a multimedia

CD to tie in with my first book, *Potatoes Not Prozac.* It was a fun idea, but I hadn't thought it through. I didn't have a clear idea of why I wanted this, what it might cost, who might buy it, whether there was a market for it, how I would fund it, how I would distribute it. I didn't do the homework, I just played with the idea. And that idea never became a reality.

Which of these is a more typical pattern for you? What do you think contributes to things working or not working? **Spend a lot of time with this exercise.** Try to tease out the things that will most support you in the diet phase. Be very concrete and specific. When I was getting ready for my own postmenopause diet, I wrote out exactly how much weight I wanted to lose. I calculated this by deciding what size clothes I wanted to wear. I knew that each size represented ten pounds, so I figured out that I wanted to lose thirty pounds or three sizes. One pound a week is a reasonable pace, so I counted out thirty weeks and set my goal to lose thirty pounds by a particular date. Then I wrote out specifically what I intended to do to accomplish that.

Annie went through this process, too, and realized that her downfall was getting food in the house and making meals. She decided to hire a personal chef but had not a clue how to go about doing it. She saw an article in her local paper about a woman starting a personal chef business. Annie called her, interviewed her, and found the woman very accommodating about Annie's dietary needs in doing the program. (Many of the recipes Annie asked the chef to make are on the www.radiantrecovery.com website, so you can use them, too, in planning your weekly eating.) The chef uses Annie's guidelines to do the planning, does the shopping for Annie, and on Tuesday makes her meals for the week. Everything is labeled and set aside in individual portions. The chef gives Annie the plan for the week. When she comes home tired and hungry, she looks at the list and pops the food in the oven. It works for her in a big way.

Entry #5

Identify the specific kinds of support for your goals that you want to have from yourself, your family, and your friends. What would it look like? Be very concrete and specific. It might be a partner or spouse who cheers you on and goes grocery shopping with you. It might be your kids agreeing not to bring candy into the house. It might be giving yourself extra time in the morning to pack a healthy lunch for yourself.

Many people tell me that the support they get on the www.radiantrecovery.com support forum is invaluable to them. Being able to connect with others at any time of the day or night reinforces the ability to stick with the program. For instance, Gail has her morning tea with her email. Her husband is thrilled with the program. He has noticed how her moods have changed from erratic and cranky to humorous and flexible. He plans special events for her and the kids and is mindful of what plans need to be made for the food. When Gail was deciding about attending a special event in another state to support her food plan, she was waffling about whether she could go. Her husband said, "Why not?" and bought the plane ticket.

You *can* find or create the support that *you* need.

Imagining Your Inside Self

You will have gathered some valuable information from doing these exercises. Let's use this growing personal awareness to get a sense of the person who lives underneath your extra pounds. First, you need to go back to any feelings of shame you have about being fat. These feelings keep you from looking at your body. Denial about how fat you are and about how you feel about being fat has kept you safe for many years, but it's gotta go if you are going to change. You need to look at how big you are. So first you are going to connect with who you are—not who you want to be or who you once were, but who you are *right now*. You are going to see your fat self the way it really is. And I will help you see your fat self with tenderness and kindness. We both know this will be hard. You have years and years of avoidance to move through. But your biochemical stability will guide you through this process.

> Because I have always struggled with shopping, I created the ritual many, many years ago of rewarding myself with a treat if I had a successful outing and actually bought something to wear! Well, you can guess what that would be . . . Mrs. Fields, anyone? Of course, an unsuccessful trip got a consolation prize. Today I had an epiphany moment—to enjoy shame-free shopping! I'm going to be there soon; I can feel it in my radiant bones.
>
> *Martha*

You notice that we did not do this exercise right off the bat. I waited until you had done enough with the food to shift your biochemistry. Your beta-endorphin levels have a huge effect on your sense of self. When beta-endorphin levels are low, you feel fat and ugly. Sugar feelings make everything much worse. When beta-endorphin levels go up, you may feel fat but you will feel mobilized. But thinking of yourself as fat and ugly keeps you stuck. Realistically assessing your body and making a plan for change is actually very empowering.

Looking at Your Body: A Shopping Exercise

Let's get started. Go into one or two clothing stores and look at the type of clothing you now buy. Let yourself really feel whether you actually like it, or whether you buy it because it's all that fits. I generally buy my clothes when I go to California, where there is a growing awareness that it's okay to wear clothes that are bigger than a size 12, so the choices are fun and interesting. But this last year I needed a new jacket and I didn't have a trip to California coming up in the immediate future, so I had to go shopping in New Mexico, where I live.

New Mexico is like Boston was twenty years ago. There aren't any clothes above a size 14 in the regular departments. This seems pretty silly, since there are great numbers of people in New Mexico who are bigger than a size 14. I had to go to the fat shops, which these days are in the regular department stores and are named euphemistically the "plus" department. When I got to the place where the fat clothes were, I reconnected to old feelings. The fat clothing wasn't the same as other clothing in bigger sizes—somehow it had lost all its shape and style. The colors were different. Basically, these were ugly clothes. These were tent clothes, ostensibly designed to hide fat, but in reality they shout to everyone which department they came from. One store had a sort of tent dress in a leopard-print fabric. This thing was so incredibly ugly, I wanted to get out of there right away! Those fat feelings were right there for me. But I was kind and tender with them, and they quieted down soon enough.

These feelings are so powerful and so deadly that we have to take the charge off them. We need to be kind to our fat self. We are going to treat him or her the way we would like to be treated. We are going to say to him or her the things we wish some salesperson would say to us: "Hey, look, I have this really gorgeous pair of slacks that really suits you. Perfect fabric, perfect color, really classy. Just right for you!" And they are.

You are going to hold this image of your real look even though you may not yet be able to get clothes in your size that look that way. You are bigger than that now. You may have to wait, you may have to find a different store that carries "good" fat clothes, but your mind needs to start holding the picture of a self that you like the looks of. Just because the clothes you can find in your area are only fat clothes doesn't mean you can't start working with the change. You need to look at where you are in order to get to where you want to be.

A Picture of the Real You

After you have gone into one or two stores where you shop now and faced and honored your fat self, you can move on to the second step of this exercise. This step is focused on discovering who you really are underneath your fat self.

When Lea was getting ready to do the shopping exercise, she was in a panic. She enlisted her best friend to go with her. She gave her the exercise to read before they went. They copied the exercise and both took it with them when they went to the store. When Lea started to panic and wanted to head for the nearest latte shop, her friend just laughed and said, "Let's go upstairs to the skinny clothes first." That kept them both focused.

Go into the boutique or department store you love the most in the whole world. Choose the department that totally suits your inside self. This does not have to be the fat department. It can be the kids' department, the men's department, or the most elegant boutique in the store.

Walk around this department. Touch the clothes. Admire them. Do not look at the sizes. Simply find colors, textures, and patterns that totally look like you. Now choose three things and take them into the dressing room. Hang them up along the wall so you can really see them. What color or colors are they? What are the textures of the fabric? What do they smell like? How do they feel against your skin? Hold them up so you can see how the color looks with your hair, eyes, and skin tone. Think about why you like these clothes. What is it that draws you to them? The cut? The style? The colors? The fabric?

Now imagine yourself wearing these clothes. Let yourself imagine that you have them on, they fit perfectly, and you feel fabulous. Let yourself imagine moving around in these clothes. Imagine where you are going in them. Let your whole body experience what it would be like to wear these clothes.

After you have done both steps of this exercise, go home and write about what you learned in your workbook. Start by writing about the fat person you met. Let yourself feel the feelings you have toward that one. Write about the feelings.

And then let yourself really feel what it is like to be the

person you want to be—the look and size and feel and energy of that person. Who is that person inside waiting for
you? Set this image in your heart. We are going to be shifting back and forth between your ideal image of the one
who is there inside and the factual image of where you
are now.

Let's Look at Your Body Size

In this exercise, you are going to take a look at how big
you actually are. Try to do this objectively. How much over
your ideal weight are you? Go stand in front of the mirror
and look. Here are the guidelines I use to define fat:

- *Really, really fat:* More than a hundred pounds over your
  ideal weight
- *Really fat:* More than fifty pounds over your ideal weight
- *Moderately fat:* Between twenty-five and fifty pounds over your
  goal weight (I sometimes refer to this as "tubby")
- *In need of trimming:* Less than twenty-five pounds over your
  goal weight

Many of us who struggle with being overweight suffer
from severe perceptual distortion. Either we look in the
mirror and see ourselves as HUGE when in fact we are
moderately fat, or we think of ourselves as moderately fat
and then are shocked to see a photograph that says we are
really fat. In many ways, our culture reinforces this perceptual distortion. Most media images of Hollywood icons
who appear attractive to some are actually anorexic. The
bottom end of sizes on the racks gets smaller as we grow
older. They didn't make size 2 thirty years ago. It is easy
enough for us to believe that these images, these smaller
sizes are the norm, but they are not. They are a cultural

distortion of what is normal and healthy. Yet even though we intellectually know they are not healthy, we have to struggle with our own idea of what to strive for. Changing the emotional imprint of what you "should" weigh will take some attentive commitment.

Take your measurements. Use your diet workbook to record your weight, and write down the measurements of your hips, your chest or bust, your thighs, your neck, and your upper arms at their widest point. I know this is going to be uncomfortable for you to do, but don't cheat. You do not have to share this information with *anyone*, but as things change, it will be a very important reference point for you. It is also going to help you desensitize the shame and disgust you have been feeling about your body. This is part of simply taking an objective look at where you are.

Now get a full-length picture of yourself. I suggest going to a professional photographer if you can afford it. They are trained to make you feel at ease. This picture is going to be very important to you. You are going to look very different in a while, and you want to mark the start of this miracle. I know this is an outrageous idea. As we get fatter, most of us avoid having our picture taken. The last thing we want to do is see the reality of how big we are. This time it's important. Get a picture. Put it in your book.

Finding Your Ideal Weight

An important fact here is to remember that we are looking for a realistic and obtainable goal. I will NEVER be a size 10, nor would I want to be. My self, my body, is not suited to that size. I am taller than average, and my ideal is to be a healthy, supple size 14. I want to be a size 14 with clothes that are comfortable and loose. The weight itself is not the marker that is most important to me. It is the weight in the context of knowing the body that fits the me of my innermost self, my soul.

Think about this exercise for a while. Talk to your friends if you are comfortable. Talk with people who have known you over time. Try on different images of yourself. See what fits best. Remember that this is a hard exercise. We have very few role models who are bigger than the models we think are the norm. But look around and notice to whom you are drawn. Observe what features or body types you like.

Even though my last name is French, I am of Irish descent. I got a copy of a magazine called *Ireland of the Welcomes*, which has all sorts of pictures of local Irish people. I looked at the pictures and decided that I have no aspirations to be Marilyn Monroe (which is probably a very good thing, since I am well over fifty), but the image of an attractive Irish mother suits me well—weighing a little above what our culture considers the norm suits my now being a grandmother. The images there helped me to see my ideal self quite well. Find something that suits you.

Now define your ideal weight. Write it here and in your diet workbook as well.

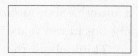

After you have done this, do a reality check. Talk with people who have a healthy body image. Describe what you feel is your ideal look and body feel. Test it with them to see if you are on track. Remember that you are seeking a body that fits who you are. Your ideal weight may be different from the culture's standard. Create what works for your body at your age in your culture. And trust your inner knowing.

Realistic Goals

Now that you have a better sense of what weight you want to be, let's figure out how to set a realistic weight loss goal for you. I want you to lose between four and eight pounds a month, no more than that. If you go faster, you will not allow your body enough time to catch up with the neuro-chemical and hormonal changes, such as increasing your overall serotonin and decreasing your hypersensitivity to big spikes of beta-endorphin.

I know you are impatient, but this piece is important. Slow is good. Slow works. Slow works for a long time. Take the total number of pounds you would like to lose and divide by five. This is the number of months you will be working on your diet plan.

Do not get spooked by how long this is. You have been fat for a long time. It didn't happen in three months. All this pain you have didn't suddenly appear in a few weeks. What you have done in the past didn't work. So this time you are going to try it a new way. A slow way. No shortcuts. No miracles. No thirty pounds in thirty days. Five pounds a month. Sixty pounds in a year. One hundred twenty pounds in two years. This way will work.

Think about the amount of time you are committing to. Let yourself really reflect on this. This is not a quick and dirty thing you are going to do. This is a major commitment of time and attention. It's a big deal.

The Scale

This may surprise you, but on this part of the plan, I *do* want you to weigh yourself regularly. You can choose how often you do this: once a week or once a month. Some people pick the first or fifteenth day of the month. I weigh myself every week on Monday morning at the same time, but what the scale says no longer determines whether I have a good day or a bad day. I no longer weigh myself in the evening to see what happened during the day. I don't obsess about it now, but I used to. The numbers I saw on the scale actually shaped my day. A pound one way or the other, and I was either elated or overwhelmed. I know that you have experienced this reality. People who do not have a problem with their weight have no clue about the power of the scale.

In this part of the plan, I want your scale to become your friend, something that reports your progress to you. And you will find that as you secure your foundation and your serotonin levels rise, you will become less obsessive about the scale. Your scale helps you be in relation to your body.

If you are very overweight, you may not be able to use a scale at home. Plan on making regular visits to a place where you can be weighed. This may be so emotionally painful for you that you want to avoid this at all costs. But what happens with your weight is going to guide you in choosing refinements to your program. If you do lots and lots of work but don't know if your weight is changing, you will not have the reinforcement of scale results. It does matter. If you don't yet have a place to be weighed without someone criticizing or reprimanding you, start working on finding one now. Ask around. Take up with other people who are very overweight and ask them what they do. If you do not have access to these kinds of resources, come to our website at www.radiantrecovery.com and ask for support.

One important function of your scale is to remind you that you need to go slowly. The ideal pattern is a loss of four to eight pounds a month, depending upon how fat you are to start with. If you end up losing fifteen pounds a month, you are going way too fast. Do *not* slip into a false elation that faster is better. That is old sugar thinking. It will get you into big trouble. Faster is not better. Faster means that your brain chemistry cannot catch up with your body. Faster means you are doing the same old, same old. Hold the image that we are reshaping your brain as well as your body and literally reforming how the molecular structure works. Taking time allows it to reform as you want it to. It works.

Changes in Your Body

As you follow *Your Last Diet!* your body is going to make more changes than just your weight. You are going to lose inches as well. Earlier I had you measure yourself very carefully. Once a month I want you to do these measurements again. Put this information in your diet workbook. You might even graph or draw the changes. If you don't do this monthly measuring routine, in six months you will have forgotten where you started.

Although this may seem inconceivable to you now, as you step into your new body you will initially want to forget your fat self as quickly as possible. Don't let this happen. After you have been doing the plan for three months, take another full-body photo. Put it in your workbook. Keep doing this every three months and write about what is happening. Schedule it in your calendar. Remember that the *Your Last Diet!* process is not designed to be dramatic; it is designed to be slow and steady. You may not see the pounds change in a dramatic way in the first three months, but you will see the other changes. You want a visual record of the miracle emerging. This process is going to change your life.

Check Your Health: The Visit to Your Doctor

Now that you have a sense of your weight goal, let's do some thinking about getting you there. Many weight loss plans tell you to diet under a doctor's supervision. I want to adapt this directive a little and encourage collaboration rather than supervision. I want you to work *with* your doctor or health care provider in getting started with your weight loss plan. *Your Last Diet!* is very safe and extremely sensible, but it is important for you to know if there are any other health issues that affect how you design your individual plan. Working as a team with your doctor or health care provider will keep you safe.

I want you to take charge of your process and how you are going to lose your weight. Many doctors still have the mind-set that to lose weight all you have to do is cut calories and increase exercise. That outdated message will only serve to reinforce your feelings of hopelessness. That's why you are going to take an active role in shaping how your doctor will support you. Reread the section on the C57 mouse studies. Mark it and take it with you when you go to visit your doctor or health care provider.

As you prepare for your visit, you may find that you are really resisting the idea of going. Some people have reported that their doctors are highly critical and very judgmental. They refuse to go see them. This is a problem that you need to look at. Why would you go to a health care professional whom you do not respect and value? Your doctor should be your biggest ally. Your doctor works for you. You pay him or her. You are purchasing a service— like any other service you might purchase—that is in support of your health and well-being. Why would you want to work with someone who is adding to your pain? If your doctor does not support you in what you have learned, find a new doctor. If you are in a managed care plan, ask to be assigned to a different doctor.

On the other hand, you may feel excited about going back to your doctor with renewed enthusiasm. You may want to share this book with your doctor. Many people have reported to me that their doctors really like my other books or that their doctor gave them the book in the first place. Physicians seem to feel that it is a reasonable plan and that the science is trustworthy. This way, you are developing support for your weight-loss process.

The Weigh-in

When you think of going to the doctor, probably the first thing that jumps into your mind is that awful moment when the doctor's nineteen-year-old assistant in a pink smock tells you to get on the scale. That is a difficult point for all of us who are sugar sensitive and overweight. Sometimes it is so awful that we actually avoid going to the doctor because we want to avoid the great weigh-in. But you do have some choices. You can decline to be weighed and give them your weight according to your scale at home. Or you can stand backward on the doctor's scale, face out, and tell the young lady in the pink smock that you do not want to know your weight. She can simply put it in the chart.

Don't skip eating breakfast on the morning of your appointment as a way of reducing the reading on the doctor's scale, okay? It won't help. I know how much we all want to cheat, but remember, *Your Last Diet!* asks that you maintain rigorous honesty with yourself. Wear your lightest-weight clothing on the day of your appointment, and take off your shoes before you are weighed. We all do this. Even I do it when I go to the doctor. Laugh at yourself.

> I went to see my doctor for a physical today. I had a pretty rigorous going-over. It went really great! The doc said he was totally blown away by my numbers and wished he could get his down there!
>
> My blood pressure was 122/80, my cholesterol was 149, and my fasting blood sugar was 77. The last time I went, my blood pressure was 140/80 and my cholesterol was 189. The only time I ever had a glucose tolerance test done, it was 199 after the four-hour test. The doc I had then said I was borderline diabetic. So needless to say, I am one happy girl tonight!
>
> *Jeannie*

Here are the things you are going to have checked. Record the results in your diet diary.

• *Blood pressure.* High blood pressure is often associated with being sugar sensitive. Remember that C57 mice are predisposed to obesity and hypertension, so high blood pressure may have kicked in simply as a result of the wiring in your body. It may have developed as you have gotten more and more overweight. Oftentimes doctors do not really know why blood pressure goes up. If yours is high, don't get alarmed. There are many, many ways to help it go down. Losing weight is at the top of the list.

If it's high, ask if you can schedule another appointment in two weeks to have it rechecked. The stress of being weighed may increase your blood pressure significantly. The dietary changes you have made in Phase 1 of your plan or are going to make in this phase may have a big effect on reducing your blood pressure.

You have time to make thoughtful, wise choices to get healthy. If you and your doctor decide that medication is the right choice for you to lower your blood pressure, make sure to learn about the medication you are taking, including its side effects. At one point I was taking some blood pressure medication and it made me really depressed. I did some research and found that this particular drug blocked the beta-endorphin receptors. It was not something my doctor had ever heard about. With his blessing, I stopped taking it and found another alternative that worked just fine. This is a good example of the partnership I want you to have with your doctor as well.

Note your blood pressure levels in your diet workbook.

• *Cholesterol.* Get measurements of both HDL ("good") and LDL ("bad") cholesterol, plus the ratio of your total cholesterol divided by your good cholesterol. Ask your doctor to take the time to explain the values.

The significance of your cholesterol levels is bigger than just one number. HDL helps the body get rid of excess blood cholesterol, and LDL causes blood cholesterol to be deposited on the walls of your arteries. (If you have a hard time remembering which is which, think of the *H* in HDL standing for "healthy" and the *L* in LDL standing for "lousy.") Unhealthy levels of cholesterol lead to arteriosclerosis, high blood pressure, and heart disease.

Traditionally, medical science has thought that high blood cholesterol was a function of eating high-cholesterol foods such as eggs and meats. However, a number of scientists more recently have looked at the role played by other dietary factors, such as sugar consumption, in your body's production of cholesterol. They found that the level of insulin in your blood (which is a function of the amount of sugars and white foods) increases the production of bad cholesterol. What you eat does affect your cholesterol—but not in the way you may have been taught. It appears that the high-cholesterol foods may not be as important as the amount of sugars and refined starches you have with them. Saturated fats and sugars together are a deadly pair, but eggs alone are not especially harmful. Many people have reported a significant change in their cholesterol readings after they took sugars out of their diet and started exercising.

Note all your cholesterol readings in your diet workbook.

• *Triglycerides.* This measurement can be taken from the same blood drawn for the cholesterol test and tells you the level of fats in your blood. Talk to your doctor about what this measurement means specifically for you. But for a start, you certainly can understand that you do not want to have fatty blood. I have a full discussion about triglycerides in the exercise chapter, "Getting Fit."

Don't forget to record your triglyceride level in your diary.

• *Blood sugar.* Be sure to have your blood tested. Many people who are overweight are either pre-diabetic or borderline diabetic. Do not get alarmed if you fall into this category. Your dietary changes are going to improve your blood sugar levels. This is one area where your doctor will be thrilled with your plan. Many, many diabetic people are in the www.radiantrecovery.com community, and their blood sugar values have improved significantly as they have gone through the program.

If you have diabetes, you will make some adaptations in your food plan. You can work with your diabetes educator to put together a plan that meshes what you are learning here with what you are learning about your diabetes. You can also come online and talk with the other sugar-sensitive diabetics who are using *Your Last Diet!* and loving its effects.

> The day before I started the program, my postprandial readings were in the high 100's. My fasting level was in the 140's. My Ha1c was 6.1. I started the program, and immediately my postprandials were down to under 140. I needed glucophage to lower my fasting level to under 126. Eighteen months later, I am completely medication free. My fasting level is consistently in the low 100s, my postprandials are always way under 140, and my Ha1c went down to 5.0.
>
> *Naomi*

As you do this groundwork, tell yourself that you are simply gathering the facts. In doing this, you are giving your body the message that this weight loss is important. You are going to spend time and money on it. You are making a commitment. What's more, the very act of letting someone else—your doctor or a new doctor—in on the process is the beginning of moving away from shame. Getting an ally sets the stage for support.

6

Checking In with Your Feelings

want you to heal. I want you not only to lose weight but to find peace, solace, and a sense of self-worth. I want you to be free of the shame, sense of inadequacy, and hopelessness you have carried for so long. I want you to heal these big feelings. As a sugar-sensitive person, you may have different kinds of feelings that affect you in powerful ways. I identify three kinds of feelings that are specific to sugar sensitivity: regular feelings, sugar feelings, and big feelings.

Regular feelings come up naturally in response to everyday life. Being mad, sad, and happy are regular feelings. They wash in and wash out in response to situations. Regular feelings usually don't last longer than about eighteen seconds. They are proportionate, clean, and responsive rather than reactive, scary, or overwhelming. They tell you that you are alive. Most sugar-sensitive people have very little experience with regular feelings before they change the food. I am sure that as you have worked this program, you have started to notice new ways of responding. When you were still eating sugars and white things, you had very little experience with regular feelings.

Your old way of eating kept you wrapped in "sugar feelings." Many of these will seem familiar and were a function of your food more than of your personality. Some sugar feelings are:

- Feeling overwhelmed
- Feeling that life is out of control
- Feeling inadequate
- Having low self-esteem
- Not being able to follow directions
- Being headstrong
- All-or-nothing thinking
- Feeling victimized
- Taking things personally
- Globalization
- Staying stuck
- Living in la-la land
- Overacting to criticism
- Being highly impulsive

Months ago, before you were doing the food, these feelings seemed real and a big part of your life. In fact, before you changed the food, you may not even have been aware of these feelings as a set of responses. More likely you felt that life got in the way of being able to feel good. Or that it was just one of those days or weeks, or you were premenstrual, or the kids were on your case. You may not have noticed that you were stuck in unhealthy patterns; you just felt fat and not able to find the right diet.

By going back and revisiting some of these feeling patterns in your food journal, you can mark the changes that have happened for you. Revisit these patterns with the care and tenderness that has emerged over the last few months. Smile at recognizing how pervasive these reactions were for you. Write in your diet workbook about how it feels to look back on these old feelings. Remember how you would have responded had anyone suggested that these things might change by changing the food.

As you read how you used to feel and react, you may be a little unnerved or embarrassed. As I looked back over my food journal and the feelings I wrote about in my diet workbook, I thought, "What if my children read this and remember those things? How embarrassing!"

The fear of being judged for our past is strong in most of us. Part of the healing is to be able to turn back to our process with clear eyes and a willingness to embrace who we were. As you read this, hold the knowledge that these responses were a function of your sugar-sensitive biochemistry. You were not a bad person; you were caught in your biochemistry and you didn't know. Your sugar feelings ran your life. And that has changed. You are on the other side. Being able to acknowledge these things will free you to move to another level.

Before doing *Your Last Diet!* I lost weight using the old diet plans, but the sugar feelings would remain. I would be thinner, I would look better, but I still struggled with the same low self-esteem, stubbornness, and impulsivity, even after many years of therapy and self-help activities. I was very insightful and understood how my family history affected my choices, yet I still felt inadequate, cranky, and out of control. But when I changed my food and started on this same plan you are now using, those feelings went away.

> I have been stable on the food since January 2000, sugar free and white-thing free, and have experienced a huge shift. First I became pleasant and playful. What a relief after years of being Mr. Hyde. Then I noticed that little things didn't really bother me. Soon big things didn't bother me. I was just steady, doing the food, observing the big stuff, and taking care of my part.
>
> About this time I began to get spooked and found myself wondering when the s—— was going to hit the fan. So I asked the old-timers on the website and they said it doesn't hit. Lo and behold, I have found that to be true for me. It is like I have good days, really good days, and great days. I never would have thought that would be possible for me.
>
> I began to notice first that my marriage has changed as if we had entered a new, even deeper, more intimate place. When sugar was in the way, clogging up the pathway, it was really hard to feel the true intimacy. My husband fondly says that I no longer have a porcupine suit on!
>
> The next huge shift has been a spiritual one. It is so wonderful to feel the connection to a higher power or God or whatever on an intense level. I really don't know if I am doing justice to the feelings. I can feel the spirit energy coursing through my body, and I LOVE it.
>
> I could sum it up by saying there is no way I would ever return to the old ways. Radiance is unbelievable, and it just keeps getting better. Everything in my life, on the outside, is the same, and yet, it all appears different.
>
> *Gail*

Let's look at what's on the other side of sugar sensitivity—the *real* states of mind underneath your sugar feelings. Let's look at the new patterns emerging. Do any of these sound familiar?

- Clear thinking
- Focus
- Responsive and reflective thinking
- Hope
- Confidence
- Ability to pay attention
- Cooperation and mutuality
- Feeling empowered
- Being realistic and appropriate
- Staying on an even keel emotionally
- Being other-centered
- Feeling mobilized and able to take action

The longer you work with your food plan, the more you will trust the balance that becomes part of your natural state. If you get slippery with your food, the old sugar feelings come back. In fact, the return of the sugar feelings is often the best clue that your food is off. You may not consciously notice your slippage at first because foggy thinking and forgetfulness reassert themselves. But you *will* eventually notice sugar feelings coming back. Whenever you do, pay attention to your food. Go back to your food journal and figure out where you are getting slippery.

Now, this may feel like a repeat of where you have been in Phase 1. You *are* going back to the same task of paying attention, but this time you're doing it with a brain that has been rewired. You will be shocked to see how different it is this time around.

Healing the Big Feelings

Once your sugar feelings and foggy or mushy brain have been healed and you are clear, calm, and steady, you have an opportunity to go back and heal the big feelings. Many sugar sensitives carry a pool of very big, very old pain beneath their fat. Sometimes you gain weight as a way to protect or buffer yourself from the intensity of feelings you cannot handle. It's almost as if you create a thick layer of fat to keep yucky stuff from hurting.

Many overweight people have experienced childhood trauma, such as physical abuse, molestation, or incest. For you, being in the body was a dangerous and painful place to be. Your cells actually became encoded with the message that being seen was too scary, so you wrapped a big, comforting layer of fat around yourself for protection. If you are someone who has had a traumatic childhood experience, losing weight can never be as simple as just making the decision to take those pounds off. Your feelings and your early bad experiences will fight you—they are encoded at the cellular level. Your body knows and remembers that being exposed is not a safe thing. So if you simply try to take it off too fast—as if you were unzipping your protective layer of fat and stepping out of it—your inside self will get scared and work very hard to protect you.

Your inside self is very powerful, and it is absolutely determined to keep you alive and safe at any cost. If it perceives that taking the weight off might endanger you, it will very effectively sabotage your efforts. Your inside self is connected to the little one who was hurt. It does not know that you are now an adult with different resources. If this is the case for you, you will need to go slowly so your inside self isn't spooked. You will honor it and work at a pace that will allow it to let you weigh less.

Sugar-sensitive people have a unique emotional hurdle to resolve as they begin to heal their biochemistry. Because you were born with naturally low beta-endorphin, your brain has learned to adjust by opening up more receptors, which makes you more affected by a beta-endorphin release than someone with normal biochemistry. When you have a beta-endorphin release, you feel it big-time. You are euphoric, your pain is numbed, and you feel on top of the world. Ironically, it's not just sugar that produces a beta-endorphin release. Stress and pain cause a release of beta-endorphin as well.

When you experience stress or pain and feel you have no control over it, it creates something science calls stress-induced analgesia. I call it going numb. This effect protects your body and your mind from harm. Big stress and big hurt create big numbing, which is *even greater* in people who are sugar sensitive because they have low levels of beta-endorphin.

The chemical effect of the beta-endorphin has an interesting by-product. Not only does it cut the pain of the stress or trauma, but it actually makes you feel as if you can cope. You feel a chemically induced sense of confidence and increased self-esteem. You do well in a crisis, remaining calm and focused—until it wears off. And then you feel restless, inadequate, and uneasy. Something is missing. Feeling as if you aren't needed or feeling bored comes from the same beta-endorphin withdrawal that takes you back to sugar.

If you continue to experience random, uncontrolled stress and you feel you can't get away from this stress, the cumulative effect makes you feel helpless. Psychologists call this state learned helplessness. Learned helplessness in C57 mice is evident when they crouch in the corner in response to new stimuli or problems. The C57 mice stop believing they can solve or get away from the problems.

In what I affectionately call the human C57 strain— sugar-sensitive people like you—I see an intriguing combination of learned helplessness and feeling like a victim, on one hand, and a striking ability to handle crisis with a sense of calm and confidence, on the other. Sugar-sensitive people can be the most incredibly skilled and competent folks in the emergency room or in fast-paced dot-com jobs. Yet when they are faced with the problem of not eating sugar, they feel inadequate, hopeless, and out of control. The people around them are baffled by the disparity between the two selves—helpless and highly competent— presenting in the same body. They often react by saying, "Why can't you just be good all the time?" But looking at this dynamic from a C57 biochemical perspective, it makes perfect sense. Shifting biochemical reactions contribute to the duality.

Doing the first phase of *Your Last Diet!* healed the biochemistry that created this contradiction. Now you can tackle your quest for drama, your crisis-seeking behavior. Do you seek out stressful situations? Do they help you numb out because on some level they make you feel safe even though on a conscious level they seem unhealthy? Are you in an abusive marriage, or do you get into relationships with people or friends who abandon you? Do you find yourself in one job after another with a tyrannical boss? Your brain and your body are trying to go back and find familiar (though painful) situations that once made you feel safe and numb because they evoked beta-endorphin.

Before you were doing the food, when your life was going well, without pain or stress, your beta-endorphin level dropped. Your self-esteem dropped, too; you became tearful and reactive, and you felt depressed and isolated. You were in beta-endorphin withdrawal, and you started craving substances (sugars and white things) or situations (painful, stressful ones) that would bring your beta-endorphin level back up again.

What's more, if you were used to the big beta-endorphin release that came from big stress or big trauma or big emotional pain (like the pain that comes with being fat), you had big withdrawal symptoms. I am not talking about just an emotional response here. This is physical; you would have had the shakes, nausea, diarrhea, and headaches; you would have been edgy and irritable; and you would have felt fat, ugly, out of control, and very, very cranky. You may have thought it was PMS or the flu or just plain ol' stress, and you would have done anything to feel better. You didn't connect this to a withdrawal that drove you like a moth back to a light bulb. You said you wanted to have a calm life, but you kept getting caught in the swirl of crisis.

On some level you learned that sugar and abuse, both of which will trigger a big new release of beta-endorphin, allowed you to function. If you took out the sugar without understanding this dynamic, you might have found yourself drifting into more drama. You would be a sugar-free drama puppy.

If your body hasn't yet learned new ways of evoking beta-endorphin, even though you are not using sugar, you may drift to the other things that in the past have worked to re-create "safety" in your brain: stress and crisis. You may seek out stressful situations not because you are

messed up, but because your body will need relief from
the withdrawal that comes when the crisis is over.

If you are not aware of this particular effect of beta-
endorphin on your brain, body, and behavior when you
design your diet plan, you will be in a world of physical
and mental hurt. If you don't understand this and you
start the diet phase, you will have a very hard time. Your
body will feel unsafe without its beta-endorphin-evoking
sweets, and it will create stress and crisis to find solace.
Your task is to understand this and to make a commitment
to consistently seek healthy ways to raise beta-endorphin
as you are doing your program.

Things such as exercise, meditation, yoga, humor,
pups, kitties, babies, dance, intimacy, and play are crucial
to the success of your diet. You want to find experiences
that create soft beta-endorphin rather than spiky beta-
endorphin. Going slowly, being mindful, taking time—all
make a difference. By nature, you like the rush of quick
beta-endorphin spikes. Unless you pay close attention, you
may find yourself working for sixty minutes on the Stairmaster, feeling fabulous, and then three hours later pick-
ing a fight with your husband to deal with coming down.

The diet part of your program demands a new level of
awareness. Getting steady with the food has taught you
how to respond to things in a different way. Now you will
apply those skills to holding feelings, to keep yourself out
of drama and in emotional steadiness as well. Make a
place every day for the soft beta-endorphin-raising activities that suit you. For example, I spend time with my pups,
the black noses, every day. Your friends may think you are
crazy to make a connection between dieting and walking
on the beach, but you know better.

You may find that you want to start or return to

therapy to heal old trauma and old patterns. The biochemical stability you now have will help you to transform
the old wounding. You will be able to change old dysfunctional patterns and create new ways of being in the world.
Your big sugar feelings will heal, and you will discover a
strong, confident self unencumbered by the old mood
swings and drama-pup behavior.

In the process of healing these feelings, being successful and effective may spook you. You may discover that
coming face-to-face with your "big" self, the one beneath
the sugar feelings catches you off guard. Many sugar-
sensitive people, especially highly successful women who
have shielded their emotional and personal power with
their sugar addiction, are surprised by the emergence of
the personal power that comes with this healing.

The old-timers in the www.radiantrecovery.com community and in *Your Last Diet!* online have talked about this
a great deal. At a recent seminar, we held what we called a
seven-step meeting—open to folks who have been doing
the full program successfully for more than a year. We
were claiming our power and authority in a way that most
of us had never done. We talked about being successful,
being transformed, moving out of crises and the diet
mentality. And we shared the joy of our skill and competence and humor. Throughout the entire meeting, every
person talked about having to move through the fear of
"being big." Martha, for instance, got a major promotion;
part of her was thrilled and another part terrified at having her power be seen. Simone was delighted to be accepted in a prestigious undergraduate program and then
had a meltdown when she grasped the implications.
Marty was named rookie of the year and was terrified that
she would never be able to do it again. After I had my first

book published, I struggled with whether it was a one-time fluke and I would never write another.

Each of these reactions was simply a different manifestation of the same sugar-sensitive fear of being powerful. Each of us talked about it with the others, who reminded us to continue with the soft beta-endorphin-evoking activities. We are all fine now and are managing our new lives very well. You will get through your own change as well!

As our food stayed steady, we no longer accepted being discounted or overlooked or ignored. We started to value who we are. We became more compassionate, humorous, and effective, and we no longer tolerated abuse, incompetence, or sloppiness. What we found in ourselves, we started to demand of those around us. And everything started to shift. The world that we used to know no longer fit who we are. All this started *before* we lost weight. We were still fat at this point, but we got mobilized to start our weight loss program.

7

Getting Fit

N ow that we have talked about feelings, I want to talk about exercise, about getting your body moving. And yes, it is something you have to do even *before* the weight loss part of *Your Last Diet!* You can use the same skills that got you steady and stable in your eating to mobilize your body.

In principle, exercise should make you lose weight because more exercise means that you burn more calories. If you burn more than you eat, you will lose weight. But for many sugar sensitives this equation hasn't worked. In fact, there is evidence that C57 mice fed a high-fat diet actually exercised more than their normal cousins and *still* gained more weight.[21] You may or may not be a couch potato, but either way your sugar-sensitive metabolism affects your weight differently than you traditionally thought it did.

If you are older than thirty, you may have attributed

your problem in getting the weight off to the metabolic and hormonal changes of aging. It is very likely true that you are not burning fuel the way you used to. But ironically, your basal metabolic rate (BMR) may be very similar to what it was when you were younger. The problem is more likely due to your decreasing ability to mobilize fat for burning and to have your fuel-burning flame hot enough.

You Are Fat and Out of Shape

Those who are most in need of exercise are either unfit, fat, or both. Getting out and exercising seems totally unrealistic. You may feel huge shame at being seen. "I could never go to the gym, Kathleen. I would be way too ashamed to be around all those athletic young people!" "Are you kidding? I can't even walk for more than five minutes without being out of breath!"

It is a vicious circle. The less fit you are, the less likely you are to exercise. The less exercise you do, the more your fitness level drops. Round and round you go, and you get rounder. But the good news is that this circle works in reverse as well. The fitter you become, the more you will want to exercise, and the more fit you will become. Take heart—the worse you are when you begin with exercise, the more dramatic the results will be.

In the past, I have been pretty laid back about exercise. I have encouraged my clients and readers to walk at least twenty minutes a day. As a dyed-in-the-wool nonexerciser, I had a worldview that focused on food rather than exercise. But my own recovery has changed that. My experience at the gym, listening to all my readers and clients, and my own scientific research have convinced me that appropriate exercise is critical to your weight loss. Exercise, like food, changes the way your body functions.

If you want to lose weight, exercise has to be part of your plan. No ifs, ands, or buts about it. Let me make the argument that convinced me. In October 1999 an article was published called "Exercise reverses peripheral insulin resistance in trained L-NAME-hypertensive rats."[24] The researcher found that ten weeks of low-intensity treadmill exercise effected a 25 percent improvement in insulin resistance. The significant factor here is low intensity. These little rats weren't working on the Stairmaster; they were simply getting up off the couch and walking. A 25 percent improvement in your insulin resistance would give you a real leg up in your weight loss plan. As you will learn in Chapter 9, insulin resistance is a key factor in gaining weight and in having a hard time losing it.

But there was even more evidence that got my attention. Another researcher showed that moderately intense exercise results in greater glucose use than restricting calories. Exercise not only burns more, it has a significant effect on the sensitivity of muscle to insulin.[25] The study showed an even more positive impact. Not only did the insulin levels drop, but total body glucose metabolism improved. The cells were sucking up the glucose and burning it because the muscles needed it for fuel and the insulin system was working more efficiently.

Having more muscle is crucial if you want to lose weight. If you are insulin resistant and overweight, you have fattier muscle tissue than your lean friends do. Their muscles are more dense. More muscle demands more fuel, which makes the body create more ways to get glucose into the cell.

In 1999, a study was published about insulin resistance

in which the researcher noted that the muscle of over-weight people "appears to be organized towards fat esterification rather than oxidation and that dietary-induced weight loss does not correct this."[26] This means you store fat rather than burn it. More significantly, it found that "dietary-induced weight loss does not correct this." *Traditional diets don't change insulin resistance.* This is why you keep getting fatter even though you diet. Insulin resistance zaps you. If you eat too much fat, your body will simply store it and add to the downward spiral. Eat too much fat, and you will get more insulin resistant and fatter in the long run. If you want to lose weight, you have to change your food and get moving. Short-term exercise is more effective than diet in enhancing insulin action in sugar-sensitive people.[27] Think about the impact of both exercise and this kind of dietary change. Reduce the foods that evoke insulin, cut the fat, and exercise!

The Hardest Part Is Getting Started

The hardest part is getting started. Feeling out of shape may overwhelm you. You may feel fat and ugly and don't want anyone to see you. You may feel you don't have money to join the gym or have no clothes to wear for exercise. You have no time, you don't want to get sweaty, or you don't want your hair to get frizzy before work. It is too much bother. You know if you do the food just right, you will lose weight and things will be fine.

It is possible for some people to lose weight just doing the food. Some, though, cannot and will never lose weight just by doing the food. You can go through every trick in the program, but if you don't exercise, not only will you fail to lose weight, you will actually gain weight even though you are doing the food perfectly. *If you want to change the lifelong pattern of dieting and gaining, you absolutely, unequivocally have to exercise.* This is not an optional part of your healing plan. It is central to it. Remember your affirmation: You will do whatever it takes to lose weight.

> After a lifetime of carrying around too much bulk, I now do a strength-training routine every morning for twelve to fifteen minutes—a split routine with free weights that has me working the nine body parts each week and one extra for abs followed by stretching. I also do twelve-to-fifteen-minute aerobic spurts every day throughout the day. Twice a week I do a one-to-two-hour bagpipe session, which can be tiring if you keep the intensity up. (I don't count daily pipe practice as strength or aerobic exercise, but hey, for fast finger twitch, there ya go.)
>
> *Connie*

Finding the Way Out

Now, I am the first to admit I am not the fitness queen of the universe. Like you, I have struggled with my exercise program and motivation. I would try something for a few weeks and then get busy and forget to exercise, reverting to my slug ways. But I found my way out of inertia. This took:

- Coming to grips with the fact that I *had* to exercise, no matter what
- Understanding why exercise was so important to my program

- Finding an exercise plan that fit my style and body
- Getting mobilized to start

As I started to learn about exercise, I discovered that most of what I had believed was erroneous or incomplete. I was stunned. I think of myself as being reasonably smart, but on the exercise line, I was a dummy. I want to take you through the process that got my attention, got me mobilized, and got me moving. It woke me up to fitness and continues to motivate me to move.

You can't move ahead in your program without moving your body. Moving your body will tell your muscles and your cells that you are serious about this. It is time for you to have a body that reflects who you really are.

Let's go back to the shopping exercise in which you remembered the look of your ideal body. Check out your shape, your clothes, and your style. Imagine your ideal body moving. What would it feel like to be in that ideal body? When I imagined my own ideal body, I felt fluid and graceful. Suzanne felt strong and grounded. Michael felt slim and surefooted. You may be excited to feel your ideal body moving, or you may get discouraged because you cannot even *imagine* an ideal body.

Don't be alarmed. Stay with me on this one. If you don't have an image, I guarantee one will come as you start to exercise. You will begin to feel your body as you move. Over time, you will feel more and more connected to your body and will be better able to imagine the power and grace of the body you want to have.

Developing an Exercise Plan

First you will get fit, and then you will lose weight. Read that again. Fit comes first, then weight loss. "Arghhhhh!" you say. "More waiting. Can't we just roll ahead with it?" Nope. Fitness first, then weight loss—just as in learning to do the food. Until you could shift from a weight loss mentality into being in relationship with your body, the program cannot work.

Your Last Diet! is not about your final diet; it is about stepping out of diet mode. The exercise is just like the food part. First you master changing your metabolism back to fat burning, and then you apply that change to specific weight loss goals. **It is slow, boring, and incredibly effective.**

Before I walk you through the changes you will make, I want to get into the why of the body changes you are going to make. This time we will start from the inside out.

Two Types of Fuel

Your body uses two types of fuel to drive your muscles: sugar and fat. It converts all you eat into these two fuel sources. Carbohydrates (sugars, white things, brown things, and green things) convert to glucose, the basic sugar fuel of your body. The fats you eat convert in your body into a whole range of fat servers called fatty acids.

Let's just focus on the fatty acids. Imagine them as tiny little tubbies swimming around your bloodstream. They want to be useful. They have their hands up to be called on. "Take me, take me," they cry. And if the muscle doesn't pick 'em, they swim off to a new site, hoping for their chance to be burned in another muscle.

When they get tired of swimming, the fatty acids go

rest in the fat cells. When they do this, they hook up in teams of three. When the little fatty acids join together, they are called triglycerides (three fats). So your fat cells are filled with little triglycerrides. When the fat cell gets full, the little fat triglycerides spill back out into your bloodstream, now joined together.

When the doctor measures your triglyceride levels, she is measuring the spillover from your fat buddies. If you have high triglycerides, your fat storage is overfull and you have lots of the buddy chains floating around. If your fat storage is full, you are fatter than your body needs. Your fat closets are overflowing.

How to Be an Efficient Fat-Burning Machine

Your body was set up to store fat because fat is the best and most efficient fuel you can get. Long ago, there were no fast foods, no grain storage silos. People ate what they caught or gathered. Food came at infrequent or unanticipated intervals. When rabbits and roots were available, people ate 'em. When they weren't, people depended on their fat stores for the fuel they needed. Getting fat was not an issue, because people burned what they stored.

Your body has long since forgotten how to be an efficient fat-burning machine. You need to help the cells remember. The cells know and will work with you if you activate the cellular memory of moving. You retrain them by exercising.

There are two types of exercise: aerobic and anaerobic. I used to think that aerobic exercise was something the Jane Fondas did at the gym: body-shaping tights, loud music, and slim young women sweating together under the tutelage of an equally slim instructor. This was not something in my frame of reference.

But this is not what aerobic exercise means. It simply means burning with oxygen. If you are gonna burn fat, you gotta have oxygen. If you get out of breath and the amount of oxygen you take in goes down, you will burn glucose, not fat. To burn fat, you need to exercise less strenuously than what we have been conditioned to think is necessary to burn calories. But you have to do it for more than a few minutes.

The problem with most couch potatoes is that our muscles have forgotten how to burn fat. They only know how to burn sugars because that is most of what we used to give them (sugar and white things). The sugars also satisfy the level of exercise we are most likely to do. You never get to the fat-burning stage.

How Long It Takes

How long it takes your muscles to move into fat-burning mode instead of fat-storage mode depends on your current level of fitness. Habitual athletes start almost immediately. In fact, they may start to burn even if they just think about exercise—their anticipation turns up the burner. Moderately fit people's fat burners ignite after about fifteen minutes of aerobic exercise. Out-of-shape people don't start burning fat until after about thirty minutes of exercise. Their muscles don't really believe them and figure they will hold out till the activity stops. Often such people are unable to create a level of intensity that burns up the glucose and looks for fat to burn.

Now, I know what you are thinking: *Thirty minutes!* The idea of exercising for thirty minutes may seem so far away from where you are now that you don't even want to start. The task seems too big. But let's back up. You are going to do a two-phase process here. First we are going to do fit, and then we are going to do fat burning. Fit means being able to walk a mile in about fifteen to twenty minutes without getting out of breath.

Realistically, when you start, you may be able to do only five minutes. You may only be able to walk one block. The important thing is simply to work with where you are and *start*. If you can only do five minutes, then walk two and a half minutes out and two and a half minutes back. But do this three times a day.

Start Walking

People who are less fit need to exercise in smaller, more manageable increments, and they need to exercise or move their bodies more often. Start walking. Whenever you walk, write it down in your food journal. Record in your food journal how long you walked, and how you felt physically and emotionally both as you did it and afterward. Sneak in a morning walk before you shower; plan ahead for a lunchtime walk. Once you master five minutes, move to seven and then to ten. After you master ten minutes, go to fifteen. After you are really comfortable with fifteen minutes of walking, shift your focus and see how far you can go in your fifteen-minute time slot. Count telephone poles, notice houses. Pay attention.

You need to pay attention because your fitness level is going to change quickly. You want the fun of knowing how much it shifts. Once you can do fifteen minutes at a reasonable pace (enough so you feel the walk has been brisk, but not so much that you are out of breath), slow the pace and extend the distance. If you are a word-smart person, write up a plan; if you are a number-smart person, make a chart. If you are a space-smart person, draw a map of your route and record the landmarks on the way. If you are music smart, take your tape player with you. If you are body smart, you are probably already walking. If you are people smart, get someone to go with you, and if you are create-your-own-world smart, use the time to enjoy your inner thoughts.

The changes in interval and intensity will alter your muscles' fat-burning ability. It's as if you are renovating an old, rusted, and dirty machine from the barn. First you clean it, scrub it with steel wool, and oil it. If you had taken it out, cranked it up, and expected it to run perfectly before you did all that work, you would have been disappointed when it jammed or froze up. But if you take care of it, you can restore it to full function. Do your exercise the way you have been doing your food: Build with small increments and pay attention.

Getting Fit

Remember that the goal for this phase is getting fit. Getting fit means reminding your body that it knows how to burn fat and wants to do it. The hardest part of this phase of the program will be the first day. Everything in you will resist starting. You will forget; you will be horrendously busy; you will have a deadline or a doctor's appointment. It will suddenly be cold, hot, or raining outside. The kids will need to go to soccer practice; you will need groceries. You will be sleepy. Anything, anything not to go on that first walk. Day one is hard beyond imagination. Day two will still be hard. But day three will bring a twinkling of change.

Marnie was a real couch potato. But she was determined to change. When she started her walking plan, she got five minutes out the door and wanted to turn around. She decided to just walk to the fourth telephone pole and back. The next day she thought she would go to the fifth.

By the end of the week, she had discovered her neighborhood. She loved seeing the gardens and the dogs as she went. It became a joy for her.

Julie's dog was getting tubby and never wanted to go anywhere except to his food dish. Julie decided to do dog walking instead of couch munching. The two of them just made it around the block. But a month later, both Julie and the pup loved their morning walk. The dog has more energy and leaps at the sight of the leash, and Julie has found her walking time to be a growing treat.

Keep at it. Check in with the forum and an online support group at www.radiantrecovery.com. Share with us what is happening. Use your support system to help you get started. But most important, get yourself moving.

Fat-Burning Exercise

Just as Phases 1 and 2 of your food plan got you ready for the diet phase, your exercise plan will progress from building a fitness foundation to adding fat-burning. Your muscles burn fat and sugar for energy, and exercise training reverses insulin resistance.[27] If you are sedentary and eat a lot, your fuel needs will be far less than what you take in. The extra will be stored as fat on your body. This part is very clear to all of you who have been overweight or still are overweight.

For people with normal biochemistry, losing weight simply requires that they eat less. Their bodies continue to burn at the same rate, but they are eating less than they burn. When the muscles ask for fuel that is not available from current supplies, the system releases extra triglycerides from the fat stores, and it is burned. These are the people for whom a reduced-calorie diet works.

For some sugar-sensitive people, this does not work.

Their muscles do not burn properly. The fat-burning mechanism isn't activated because they are not exercising. The longer they maintain their couch potato status, the less efficient their fat burning becomes. Insufficient fat burning coupled with insulin resistance is a double whammy. Not only do the muscles burn fat inefficiently, but they also have a hard time getting the fuel they need. They are damped down by the insulin resistance. Insulin-resistant couch potatoes are unlikely to lose weight adequately even if they cut calories and exercise moderately.

Some sugar sensitives who cut way down on their food intake and exercise vigorously lose weight initially but then plateau. The scale will not budge further. They too are inordinately frustrated because they are not getting the results they want. They do not understand that they are not getting enough to eat to match the level of exercise, and so their bodies are holding on to everything they can. Sometimes these people actually need to eat more to jump-start their weight loss.

The answer for all these folks is essentially the same: The weight loss equation must be tailored to your own specific biochemistry. "Eat less, exercise more" is a recommendation for a very small number of sugar-sensitive people. The best option is a new equation that says:

- Eat the right amount of the right foods at the right time for your body.
- Exercise at the right level of intensity to get the results you want.

Fitness for Fat Couch Potatoes

When a fat couch potato starts getting fit, there is very little fat burning going on. The couch potato's body simply

burns the sugar in the blood and never gets around to using up fat stores. You may think you have to exercise hard,
work up a sweat, and be out of breath in order to burn fat.
This is not true. The more you are out of breath, the less
you are burning fat. Breath brings oxygen. Oxygen burns
fat. Exercise as hard as you can without getting out of
breath so you don't lose the fat-burning oxygen coming
in. The best aerobic (oxygen-using) exercise has three
major parts.

- **You go the ideal amount of time.**
- **You breathe deeply but are not out of breath.**
- **You use big muscles like your thighs and butt (they burn more).**

The ideal amount of time means you can exercise and
not feel as if you are going to die. When I started my own
exercise program, I started walking. I walked twenty minutes for about a week or so and then expanded the time.
My walking routine was hardly joyous, but it was consistent. After three weeks I was walking a mile in that time.
Surprisingly, in another two weeks I could walk the same
mile in less time. I was getting fitter without realizing it.

My Experience at the Gym

About this time, I decided to get a membership in my local gym. I chose a place that is family oriented, with people of different ages and shapes, not just the young,
vigorous, shapely ones strutting around. I decided to work
on the cross-country ski machine. At the time, I didn't
know it was the most intense option. I just knew that I had
loved to cross-country ski as a young woman.

So I started. After five minutes my legs were screaming
and wobbly, I couldn't breathe, and I thought I would

pass out. I was shocked. I knew I was out of practice (that means out of fitness), but the degree of it stunned me. But I went again the next day, telling myself, "Just get to five minutes, Kathleen. That's all you have to do." Only one week later five minutes was easy, so I started to increase the time by one minute a day. By the end of the month I was doing thirty minutes a day, without pain and without being out of breath.

Around the second week, I realized that a good part of hanging in there was finding a way of coping with my boredom. The gym has TVs, and if you bring your own earphones, you can listen to whatever channel is most interesting. I soon learned about daytime TV and that finding an interesting topic on the afternoon talk shows made the thirty minutes fly by. No one had ever talked to me about the boredom of exercise, but I assure you that you need to consider it in your plan if you want to be successful.

Continuing

Regular, constant aerobic exercise is the way to go. Nothing flashy, no drama, no fancy routines. Just regular, boring ol' "do it." But the most extraordinary thing will happen. One day, unexpectedly, you will *feel* the fat burning kick in. For a couch potato, it is an awakening experience unlike anything you have felt in years, maybe in many years. You will *know* the feeling. Everything starts to stream. Maybe the little triglyceride buddies are swimming. Maybe they are singing. It is as if your body wakes up and says, "Yes!"

I have often said that if a person can get one week steady on the food, she will always go back to it. There is a body memory of things feeling right. I think the same thing is true with exercise. When we diddle with it, or when we never push ourselves to the fit state, we never feel that *yes*. We remember the boredom, or we remember feeling terrible because we pushed too hard too fast and didn't get results. No wonder we drop it so quickly.

Keep working at the aerobic (remember *oxygen*) program. In fact, maybe you should think of it as your oxygen program. Every day. Thirty minutes. And if you are a mega couch potato, make that thirty minutes twice a day and watch those triglyceride buddies swim into your muscles to be burned.

Weight Training

The next piece is specific muscle training. You want to have a higher proportion of muscle because muscle is what burns fat. Sugar addicts are big but flabby. Converting fat to muscle is the ideal plan. More and better muscle will make the cumulative program far more efficient.

Weight training works. Go to the gym. Get a trainer who likes people like you. The ones who do rehab training are often kind and patient and will offer enormous support for your program. If the first trainer you get isn't up to speed or is bored with your program, change trainers. Find someone who teaches you how the muscles work, where they are, which muscles to exercise in which sequence. Don't be fooled by glitz; insist on someone who knows about fat burning. You want to understand exactly what is happening. This is *your* body, and it deserves your attention.

Aim for exercises that allow you to do twenty reps (repetitions) without strain. If you master a given weight level, increase it incrementally.[28] Choose the weight level that allows you to get to twenty reps with a tired but not injured muscle. You want to make the muscle work just to the point before it begins to release lactic acid (which produces a burning sensation in the muscle—not to be confused with the fat-burning process). This will also increase the level of beta-endorphin in your bloodstream and will enhance the feel-good effect of the workout.[29] If you can't lift it more than six times, it is too heavy. If you can lift it thirty times, it is too light. Your body doesn't lie. Listen to it.

If you start your gym routine with a series of stretches and then do weights and your aerobic training, you will maximize your fat burning. The weight training will burn off the glucose, and by the time you start to cycle, row, or walk on the treadmill, you will be burning fat. But remember to stay at the level where you are not feeling muscle burn. If your muscles start to feel as if they are burning, it means they are releasing lactic acid and not burning fatty acids.

Too Busy to Go to the Gym?

Many people tell me that they are way too busy to get to the gym because of kids, family, work, and other commitments. I have been there and said that. What you have to do is to schedule exercise time as if it were the most important activity of your schedule. The kids can wait, billable hours can wait, and your friends can come with you. Go to the gym. You will discover the miracle of time expanding. Exercise and you will have more focused energy than you ever dreamed of.

If you think you can't afford the gym, shop around. Try the YMCA or YWCA. See if your local high school or community college has a weight room that local residents are allowed to use. Work something out with a local hotel with a fitness room. And if the cost is still out of your range, go to the library and find some books on weight training. I love the *Weight Training for Dummies* book. Many people like *Strong Women Stay Young*. Look for books that suit your style. Use soup cans as weights for your arm exercises. Get creative. Exercise equipment can easily be found at yard sales or flea markets. Get a stationary bike or a rowing machine and use the machine while watching TV. Dust your bicycle off, go hiking, or learn to use in-line skates. You will be burning fat. Go on a quest. And keep walking while you are getting ready to do the more intense exercises.

You Can Overtrain

Another important issue for weight loss is overtraining. Exercise breaks down the muscles. If you exercise vigorously and do not rest adequately, your muscles have no time to rebuild and become stronger. If you don't have sufficient rest, the muscles can't help you in the fat-burning process. They will be busy trying to recuperate rather than help. The rebuilding time is essential.

Some sugar sensitives become compulsive exercisers rather than couch potatoes. They use the Stairmaster for an hour every day. They generate huge amounts of beta-endorphin by the intensity of their exercise and then feel terrible when they get a withdrawal crash. They think that the exercise is the only thing that keeps them sane. They do not realize that what they think is comforting them is actually creating the problem. If your body cannot clear the effect of the exercise, you do not get the same benefits.

The Total Program

After all of this, what will your exercise plan likely look like? You will start with the get-fit process and work up to walking thirty minutes a day. You just work on this in little chunks. Don't spook yourself about how impossible it seems. Start with five minutes and one block or five minutes and two hallways—tiny little chunks in the beginning. The daily routine will get set, and then you will start to think about your weight loss program.

The first phase of weight loss exercise is introducing more vigorous aerobic exercise that mobilizes big muscles and makes demands on the muscle system. You will choose a specific kind of fat-burning exercise that fits your style. It might be walking outdoors or on the treadmill, using the Stairmaster or the elliptical trainer, rowing or using the cross trainer at the gym. Whatever you choose, you go through the same process of making small incremental increases that build to the fat-burning stage over time. You start with five minutes and build to thirty. It make take a month or even two, but if you do this every day, you'll get there.

The second phase of your weight loss exercise adds in weight training for big muscles, little muscles, funny muscles, and sleek muscles. This is weight training. You can do it either at the gym, using the weight machines or free weights, or at home with the help of a book from the library. Jan hired a personal trainer and goes to the gym three times a week. She is fifty-nine years old and beats out the thirty-year-olds every time. She got an award for being the best client of the month for her commitment and diligence. When she started she thought she would die. Now these sessions are the highlight of her week.

Even under the fat, you will be mobilizing those muscles to remember how to burn fat. They will get stronger and more interested in your fat burning as you work them. You may not get buns of steel right away, but you will start the fat burning. Learn the different muscle groups and how to exercise each one. When you do weight lifting, build to twenty repetitions. Once you can easily do twenty, make the weight heavier. Rest briefly and do it again. Try for twenty repetitions of each muscle group three times in a row. Breathe in while lifting and breathe out while lowering the weight. Raise the weight quickly and lower it slowly. Do your program every other day so your muscles can rest, rebuild, and grow. If you want to lift weights every day, rotate the muscle groups so they can rest. Many people do their lower body one day and their upper body the next. My trainer suggested doing a front/back split instead. I like it much better. I do the muscle groups on the front of my body one day and those on the back of my body the next. Somehow this seems more connected to me. It gives the muscles an opportunity to rest but allows me the fun of working out every day.

You are on your way! You may have started getting fit as a way to enhance your weight loss, but something else is going to creep in. You will want to move. Maybe you'll have the urge to break into a jog, even run halfway around the track; maybe you'll feel like putting on your swimsuit and going for a swim. You may go looking at the in-line skates in the fitness store rather than cakes in the bakery. You'll discover little but surprising changes—I promise. You are on your way!

Doing the Diet

You may have come to this section first, blithely ignoring the other chapters. If so, you aren't supposed to be here yet! If you do this chapter first, the program won't work. If you do this chapter first, it will be just like any other diet you have ever done. Actually, it will be worse, because this part is sort of boring. You will feel cheated and misunderstood. You will decide that I don't understand what things are like for you with food and weight. I caution your impetuous, sugar-sensitive little soul: Don't set yourself up for failure. Please, please, please start by doing the homework—Phase 1—before you try this. There is too much at stake to rush to the end first. So if you aren't supposed to be here, go back to the beginning and start with Step 1.

If you come to this chapter *after* doing the foundation and getting steady, after living from that place for a while, and after learning how food and steadiness affect your own body, I guarantee things will change. You will lose weight. This phase of the plan won't seem overwhelming or too difficult. It really is simply an adjustment of your food and exercise: nothing more, but everything different.

For those of you coming to this chapter having done all the homework, you *know* this plan is different from every diet you've been on in the past. Doing the foundation work before starting the diet part has been critical. You learned why just saying no to sweets will not work for you, and that you need to go slowly and heal your biochemistry *before* losing weight. We rewired your brain so you *can* say no—with power, authority, and a sense of being in charge. This ability didn't happen simply by deciding, and it didn't develop overnight.

Because we have done all this work in preparation, you are feeling confident and ready to start the weight loss phase of your program. The foundation work you have done has stabilized your blood sugar volatility, increased your serotonin levels, stopped the beta-endorphin priming that comes from sugars, and increased your levels of beta-endorphin. The weight loss process is simple and straightforward. Creating that firm foundation we have been talking about in the earlier chapters has gotten you to a unique place. You have done the hard part. The weight loss is simply a refinement of the steadiness that is so familiar now.

The weight loss phase has more to it than simply getting on with your diet. As you learned to heal your sugar sensitivity, you went through a sequence of learning about the issues, trying some new behaviors in a logical and sequential way, and reflecting on your experience. You will be using this same approach in the weight loss phase. How much you weigh and how easily you will lose weight depends on how sensitive your body is to the insulin you produce, how well you burn fat, whether you have any food allergies, and how your thyroid is working. It also depends on how fat you are, your emotional readiness, your style of making changes in your life, your prior experience with weight loss, your skill in following the plan, your ability to stay steady with the foundation of the program, your exercise level, and your support network.

Successful weight loss requires that you understand these components and sort out which apply to you and to what extent. Please note that I have **not** included your willpower, your commitment, or your self-discipline. I am assuming you are committed. You would not have bought this book and done the work you have done up to this point if you weren't. Willpower and self-discipline are not critical factors. They are a function of your biochemical state; you have seen them emerge as you do the food, and they will continue to build. By doing the foundation work, you have experienced exactly what I am talking about. Everyone has a similar core weight loss program, but you refine it depending on your unique body needs.

Your body will guide you. **The standard for the plan working is whether you are losing a pound or two a week.** If you are already losing a pound or two a week (not more, not less), then simply keep doing what you are doing. If not, then you will shift your food and your exercise until you do. You will do this progressively. First you do the diet food plan, which is simply a refinement of what you are already doing. If you are not yet losing weight with it, then you look at your insulin resistance and tweak your plan accordingly. If you are still not getting results, then you look at how your thyroid is functioning. And finally, you will look at whether you have any food allergies.

At this point in your process, I am assuming that you

have completed the seven steps of Phase 1, you have an exercise plan in place and are doing it, you are emotionally ready to start, you know your own style of making change, and you have a support network in place.

To lose weight, you will design a plan to work with your style, your body, and your emotional readiness. You will not have exactly the same plan as someone else, nor will yours follow the same timing. You may have some residual diet expectations and want to be told exactly what to do with the food groups, the blocks of protein, fat, or carbohydrate. You may still want calorie or fat gram guidelines and to be told what to eat on day 1 and day 2. Or you may go to the other extreme and want to do it entirely your way, figuring that because I am telling you to develop a plan to suit your needs, you should ignore the guidelines of the foundation and simply make up your own plan from scratch. None of these approaches will work.

By now, I am sure you realize that sugar-sensitive people either do not like rules at all or want to be told what to do every step of the way. We are all-or-nothing people, bouncing back and forth between being all over the place and being inappropriately rigid. You have learned that you need a rhythm that allows you to have the best of both options—to have enough structure so you feel safe and directed and enough flexibility so you are pushed to define *your* needs and rhythm. Because you have been doing the food and know the drill for stability, you are no longer frantic and are starting to enjoy this program. You have your weight goal, and you know it will take a week for each pound or two. Now you are going to design the actual food plan for the process. Let's review where you are now.

YOU ARE STEADY WITH YOUR FOUNDATION

- You are keeping a daily food journal and using it as a supportive tool in talking with your body.
- You are eating three meals a day with protein at each meal.
- You eat that little potato every night before you go to bed.
- You have shifted your carbohydrates from white things to brown things.
- You have completed your sugar detox.
- You are drinking lots of water.

YOU HAVE DONE ALL THE PREPARATORY EXERCISES

- You have done the preparation exercises and written down your experience in your diet notebook.
- You have actually gone back and read what you wrote, thought about it, and incorporated it into your life.
- You know your style; you know which intelligences are strongest, and you can draw strength from them.
- You are not concerned about the areas where you are less strong; you know how to plan for them and not be spooked by them.
- You have been to the clothing store and are connected to the colors, styles, and possibility of the new you.
- You have been to the doctor and have gotten the baseline information and written it in your diet notebook.
- You are raring to go.

YOU HAVE STARTED EXERCISING

- You have worked out an exercise plan that suits your body and lifestyle, and you are actually doing it.
- You are doing both cardiovascular (aerobic) exercise and weight training.

YOU HAVE REFLECTED ON HOW YOUR FEELINGS SHAPE YOUR EATING

- You understand your behavioral patterns and how emotional eating factors into how much you weigh.
- You have identified whether old trauma or messages interfere with your ability to lose weight; if they are there, you are taking steps to heal them.
- You have built a support network for losing weight, so you have sympathetic, caring people who are excited about the plan and willing to help you do it. If you have people around who attempt to sabotage your plan, you have sorted out strategies for disengaging from their negative energy.
- You know what you want and you have a system in place to get it.

In *Your Last Diet!* you will be eating according to the plan you have worked out for your body. *You* are the expert on this diet. My job is to provide you with clear, reasonable information so you can make informed choices. If you are not losing weight the way you feel you should, you will have the tools to ask the right questions and make the adjustments that will get you moving again.

This kind of healing is not about doing it and never turning back. It is a living, working plan. Sometimes you will do better than other times. Sometimes you will slip and slide. Sometimes you will do fabulously. All who do the plan have done both. This is natural and is actually part of what helps you to make the changes in your food that will last long after you have finished doing a diet. Slipping teaches you about your body and your brain chemistry. Learn from it. Hang in there and do the plan despite your slips, and this will change you. Commitment creates a plan that endures. I want you to lose weight, too, but something even bigger is happening, and you will know it in every part of your being. This miracle is bigger than food.

I plan to learn from this slip and not let it conquer me. I had a long period of doing this program well (though not perfectly), and it enabled me to see that the real problem stemmed from eating "just a little" of the food I knew could get me into trouble. I did this because I was not attending to keeping my serotonin and beta-endorphin levels up. This of course led to my body chemicals going amok, and off I was into the land of more than "just a little."

I'm in a relapse now, so I looked back in the journal and saw that I got back onto foods that get me out of biochemical balance. So I had my protein for breakfast again today. Tonight I intend to plan out my week's menu, go back to my gym routine, and weather out the detox. Hopefully it won't be as intense as it was before. I am in the process of creating a new history for myself—one in which I heal at a cellular level.

Laura Rose

The Diet

You are going to do these basic things in your diet:

- Adjust the amount of food you are eating so your portion sizes work for you
- Change your proportion of browns and greens
- Change the amount and kind of fat you eat
- Increase your exercise

• Keep working with your emotions and any fears of being strong, powerful, and successful

This is the diet. Compared to the steps you've already taken, it's pretty simple. Sort of anticlimactic, yes? It probably sounds like almost any other diet you have ever done. This is the irony of those diet recommendations. In many ways, there is truth to them. In fact, most of every diet you have ever done has a piece of the true diet story embedded in it. Atkins is right on the money with cutting out sugars, Sears understands how to control insulin spiking, the Eadeses are very clear about the role of protein, and the Hellers hit the mark with carbohydrate addiction. But without understanding how sugar sensitivity shapes the impact of each of these, you have not been able to put things together the way you now can. Now you can see the role your brain plays. It is your biochemistry and not your willpower that has gotten in the way.

Now, for Losing Weight . . .

Let's start with how much to eat. Part of the trick to losing weight is to eat the amount of food that is right for your body's needs. Some sugar sensitives will need to eat less and some will need to eat more in order to lose weight. That sounds sort of strange, doesn't it? Why am I not telling you to eat a certain number of calories based on your weight, height, and age?

I know you want it to be simple. I know you want to know exactly what to do and have it succeed the first time out. But it doesn't work that way. The whole premise of this book is for *you* to sort out what works for you. Finding the right amount of food for your body is critical. If you are eating a lot, even though the food is well balanced for your sugar-sensitive body, you may need to eat less. You are very familiar with that drill. But it is critical that you understand you are not to make the assumption that less is better in all cases—you must ask your body. To do this, you must think not only in terms of calories, fat grams, and counting. You must understand that there is an ideal amount that will allow your body to burn more than your food intake. But as simple as it sounds, this can be tricky.

There are two major approaches to this phase of your program, counting and estimating. I have worked with many, many people over time and have seen that there really are two core groups—those who love to count and feel empowered by it, and those who do not—and never the twain shall meet. I am not a counter, although I did try it and I just couldn't do it. As soon as I start count- ing, it feels like a drag and I hate the whole plan. I don't count, and I have a plan that works for me. But I also honor the power of counting for those who count. I am going to speak to both options. You can choose the one that suits you.

Let's speak to the numbers folks first. Suggesting that you count is a big step on my part. For years and years and years I have told people *not* to count. I *still* say don't count for the first seven steps of *Your Last Diet!* Counting early in your recovery is a recipe for disaster. It only reinforces old and unhealthy patterns. But I have come to see that if it is done by a person who has laid the foundation, counting can be a valuable tool for creating a workable food plan, because you now have the biochemical balance, the skills, and the mind-set to manage counting in a healthy way.

I'm a numbers person. I think they are beautiful! I have a close personal relationship with my ten-year old HP calculator, which does absolutely everything. And don't even get me started on number theory!

I have had a diet consciousness in the past, so now I tend to stay away from calculating as far as my food is concerned. And since my food is steady and things are going well, why bother with anything like that?

On the other hand, if I start to have problems with the food, I'm willing to do whatever analysis it takes to figure it out. Anyway, it's nice to know there are sugar-sensitive number lovers out there.

Sally

Now, there is one very big dilemma in my recommendation to count. The software currently on the market to do this is limited in what it can give you. It is either very user friendly with an incomplete database or it has a great database and is impossible to use. Check the website at www.radiantrecovery.com for the latest information on which software I recommend. For now, you will have to do the best you can. Essentially, you are going to build an equation that will get you to that weight loss of one or two pounds per week. Get a baseline by actually calculating what your current food plan consists of. You need to find out how many calories you are having and how they break down into protein, fat, carbohydrates, sugars, and fiber. You will also want to see how your fats break out into saturated and unsaturated and what proportion of omega-3 and omega-6 fatty acids you are having. The software you use should allow you to enter your age, sex, activity level, and current weight to establish the number of calories needed to maintain your body weight. It will also allow you to set a goal weight and a projected weight loss of one or two pounds per week to see how many calories a day will work for you.

As you use this information, remember that it is calculated on traditional dietary values and ratios. It is not taking your sugar-sensitive body into consideration. You will need to do that by using the counting information to see what works for you. For example, the software may tell you that you can eat 1,900 calories a day and lose a pound a week. If you plan your meals around it for a month and find you are losing three pounds a week, your addictive nature will be thrilled. However, this kind of thinking will take you right back to diet mentality—the very thing you have been working to put aside for all these months. Your task will be to stay in your recovery self and look at the rest of the equation to see what you might add in order to get to the goal of one or two pounds a week.

The Stable Protein Flame

If you are like me and not into counting, simply work with your existing food plan and adjust it as I show you. Keep the level of protein you are having at breakfast, lunch, and dinner absolutely steady at 0.4–0.6 grams per pound of your body weight per day. Each meal should have one-third of that amount. (If you are over 250 pounds, remember to use the 250-pound mark as your base.) Do not skimp on protein. When you are in the weight loss phase, you absolutely must pay attention to the regularity of your meals and the type of protein you eat. In many ways, protein stability is the heart of your plan. It is why we have waited for you to master the routine before shifting into this phase. Still, we are doing *not* a high-protein diet, but a consistent moderate-protein diet.

Use hard-core protein—eggs, meat, poultry, and fish. Don't use peanut butter as a protein source. The fat-to-protein ratio is so high, it isn't worth the trade-off. Don't use yogurt, either. Rely on things you can hold in your hand. If they ooze out, don't use them. Oily fishes like salmon are tops. You may want to have salmon two or three times a week because they are high in omega-3 fatty acids. Many of the large discount stores like Costco and Walmart now carry excellent salmon steaks or filets. Go ahead and get a big piece, cut it into individual servings, freeze them, and use as needed. When you freeze them, put them in individual plastic containers, cover them with water, and tightly close the lid. This will prevent freezer burn and reduce odor when you thaw them. If you are a vegetarian, keeping the protein steady is even more crucial for you; use tofu, tempeh, and proteins such as lentils or garbanzo beans.

The protein is what your body will use to sustain your metabolic fire. If you skimp on the protein, you won't get the "hot" effect you are seeking. To lose weight, your body has to burn hotter and longer. Science calls your burn rate thermogenesis. I call it heating up. Let's start with a metaphor to explain your special sugar-sensitive metabolism. Think of your body as an oven. To make energy, you need both heat and something to burn. I live in the Southwest, so I like to use the image of a horno, a beehive-shaped oven made from adobe. Imagine that you need to choose the best fuel for your task. Your choices are newspaper, pine, oak, or mesquite. As you know, each will make a very different type of fire. The newspaper will burn quickly, with a lot of heat but no staying power. The pine will crackle and pop with a lot of resins and give you some heat for a short cooking job, but it will burn up quickly. The oak will burn smooth and hot and long. The mesquite will generate an even more intense, slow heat, and a hot flame.

Imagine that carbohydrates serve as fuel for the fire we are going to build in your body. The complexity of the carbohydrates will determine how long and how hot they will burn. Sugars are like paper. White things are like pine. Brown things are like oak. Green/yellow/red things (vegetables) are like mesquite. Brown, green, yellow, and red things are all complex carbohydrates. The slower and more complex the carbohydrate, the more intense the heat. If you want to burn hotter, you need to use the kind of fuel that generates the most intense heat. The hotter the heat you need and the longer you need it to last, the more careful you have to be about how you get the fire started. Protein is the flame that will ignite your fuel. A little flick of a match will ignite newspaper, but it won't get an oak log burning. And without a hot flame, mesquite will only smolder, not burn. It is the combination of the hot flame of the protein and the complexity of the carbohydrate fuel that creates the long and effective burn you want in order to lose weight.

You need to eat more of the foods that give you the hottest burn. Those foods are slow carbohydrates, the slowest you can find: high-fiber brown things; green, red, and yellow vegetables. Lots of vegetables. Mix your oak with mesquite for the best effect. You need to light your fire with plenty of protein so it will heat up the slow carbohydrates cooking in your body. Since the protein and complex carbohydrates dance together, you will also increase your protein intake.

Eating enough ounces of protein at every meal is going to take focus and attention. You will have to prepare for it. You will have to think through what you are going to eat and when. You will need to make sure you have what you need on hand. You do not want to let the fire burn out. If there's no fuel, there's no burn, no weight loss. When you were doing Phase 1, you had more latitude. The diet phase (Phase 3) means paying attention.

Making an extra portion at dinner makes it easier to have lunch ready for the next day. You cannot skip a meal when you are in diet mode. You can't eat on the fly. You can't forget to eat, then grab something two hours later. Paying attention and eating at regular intervals are crucial. I have found the "make it at dinner and save some for the next day's lunch" trick really useful for staying with the plan.

By now you should be able to translate food weight in ounces into grams of protein. If you are still fuzzy about how to do this, either get a little book to tell you the protein amounts for the foods you eat or use a software program to calculate the exact number of grams in each food. Remember: protein at the core, and slow carbohydrates as the garnish!

Carbohydrate Fuel

Eat two to three cups of slow carbohydrates at every meal. Adjust the total amount to your current body weight. If you are larger, eat more; if you are smaller, eat less. The recommendation for two to three cups covers people who weigh from about 150 to 250. Remember that those of you who are currently over 250 will be planning for a 250-pound body. If you weigh 290, you will not be having more than three cups. If you weigh 125, you will not be having less than two cups. Mix green and brown carbs. Vary the ratio of brown things to green things in these three cups to find the best combination for you.

Many people start their healing with a higher percentage of browns, such as two-thirds browns and one-third greens, and then shift more toward one-third browns and two-thirds greens. Your software counting program won't differentiate between a brown and a green and a yellow. It is essential that you have some browns with every meal. Do not go below a half cup of browns per meal. Do not get excited and think that if some veggies are good, all veggies are better. The ratio is important.

The weight loss plan has a higher percentage of greens to browns than the stability plan you are used to. Ideally, you will include some greens at every meal. However, I am aware that some people cannot stand the idea of vegetables at every meal.

Vegetables at breakfast may seem un-American. Think of the overall balance of your carbohydrates as a daily process rather than a process for each meal. If you don't like the idea of veggies for breakfast (which you can chop up and sauté or mix with eggs or tofu), use brown things (such as oatmeal, brown rice, or whole grain toast) and protein at breakfast, and then have protein with proportionately more veggies for lunch and dinner. Lunch and dinner should always include a small portion of browns.

Keep eating the evening potato with skin. You may want to move to a smaller one as you are more and more steady. But keep eating it. You may continue to have something on the potato, but while you are in the weight loss phase, you will want to pay attention to the amount and kind of fat you are using. I will write more about this in the fats section.

Vegetable Abundance

If you are not a veggie person (or maybe even if you are), at first glance this plan may seem sort of serious. I mean, after all, is there anyone in the world who wants to eat vegetables night after night? If you frame your vegetable thoughts in this way, it will indeed be boring and quite possibly grim. But there is an alternative. There are hundreds and hundreds of vegetable cookbooks just waiting for you to find them. I recently went to the bookstore on your behalf. There was a whole section of books on veggies and another whole section for vegetarians (a place to find more helpful hints). These books have thousands of interesting things to do with your green and red and yellow friends. There are even hundreds of recipes for spinach! There is an awesome site for vegans at www. abbeysvegetarianrecipes.com.

For example, you can mix eggs and cheese (protein) with your spinach and come up with a yummy spinach soufflé (made with whole wheat flour, not white flour). Or you can grill those veggies and think you died and went to heaven. The most important thing is trusting that it will be okay. Even if you don't like veggies, we will find a way around it. I promise.

And yes, you can add some olive oil or salad dressing to your veggies. The addition of oil, salad dressing, or sauce (unless it is made with white flour or contains sugar) to your vegetables is a very important part of this plan. This is not intended to be a no-fat plan. Nor is it intended to go all out with the oil. Pay attention to the amount of fat you are using. Remember your body needs essential fatty acids to function. Choose your fats wisely and pay attention to the type of fat you have. Olive oil, sesame oil, and flaxseed oil are all good alternatives, but do not use corn oil because it is so high in omega-6 fatty acids. I will talk more about this in the fats section.

Do not be fooled into thinking that if you do the veggies and also do no-fat, you will be creating the ultimate weight-loss program. Wrong. You will only be creating one cranky sugar-sensitive person! Moderate amounts of the right kinds of fat will not only help raise your beta-endorphin level, make you feel better, and help you stick with the plan, but actually enhance your weight loss. Eating all these veggies is not exactly the most exciting thing in the world, so you gotta have some fun here, but judiciously using good fats can enhance both your health and your attitude.

This is *not* a low-carbohydrate food plan. Your body needs carbohydrates to function. Do not be tempted to cut carbs and think the plan will work better. Remember the oven. We are looking for a long, hot burn. If the flame (protein) has nothing to ignite, it doesn't matter how hot it is. There is a very large push in the diet world to do high protein and very low carbs. This equation does jump-start weight loss by the metabolic changes it creates. It feels glamorous, it is quick, and it seduces you into thinking it is a great way to go.

Often new dieters will say to me, "I am just going to do the low-carb thing until I lose weight, and then I will do

Your Last Diet!" This is the equivalent of saying, "Let me go disturb my body metabolism and add to my imbalance for the sake of losing ten pounds, and then I will spend more time, more energy, and more effort in repairing it with your program." As you might guess, I don't think this is the best option. It is not healthy, and the long-term effects can be very problematic. Do slow carbs rather than low carbs. You will get the best of all possible worlds with your weight loss plan.

You get to choose the ratio of green things to brown things that you will eat. You are going to ask your body and your scale what mix works best for you. There is no diet sheet because you are going to write the plan best suited for your body. And you are going to adapt it as you go. You are going to continue the miracle of learning, exploring, and planning you have already done over the past months. Your journal and your scale will guide you. The very things that used to tyrannize you will become your friends in the process.

Using the Carbohydrate Continuum to Build Your Plan

The carbohydrate continuum will show you the relative burn value of various carbohydrates. You will not see proteins on this list, only carbohydrates. Proteins are so much more complex than carbs, it would require extending the page out another three feet to fit them on a relative continuum.

The simpler carbs are on the left and the complex carbs are on the right. As you move from left to right, you will see the carbs that take longer for your body to metabolize. Alcohol is listed here because even though pure alcohol has no carbohydrate in it, many alcoholic beverages, such as wine and beer, also contain a high percentage of sugars because of the rest of the liquids that have not converted to alcohol. The sugars compound the beta-endorphin effect of the alcohol. I think of beer and wine as liquid sugar.

When you started this food plan several months ago, you were probably eating carbohydrates in this kind of proportion:

ALCOHOL	SUGARS	WHITE THINGS	BROWN THINGS	GREEN THINGS
◆	◆◆◆◆	◆◆◆◆◆◆		◆

In laying the foundation in Phase 1, you have shifted your carbohydrates to the right. You took out alcohol, sugars, and white things.

ALCOHOL	SUGARS	WHITE THINGS	BROWN THINGS	GREEN THINGS
			◆◆◆◆◆◆	◆◆◆

When you move into the weight loss phase of your plan, you are going to choose how fast you go to achieve your loss rate of one or two pounds a week. You can continue what you have already been doing.

Some sugar-sensitive people find that the seven steps of the foundation phase are all they need to lose weight consistently and steadily. Their bodies burn hotter naturally, so the shift to the right side of the carbohydrate continuum that is inherent in the foundation phase is all they need to do in order to lose weight. Sometimes, however, these folks find that the foundation helps them lose weight for a few months and then they level off. When that happens, I recommend that they shift to less brown and more green, like this. You will notice the ratio is one-third browns to two-thirds greens for this person.

ALCOHOL	SUGARS	WHITE THINGS	BROWN THINGS	GREEN THINGS
			♦♦	♦♦♦♦

How Fruit Fits

You may have noticed that I haven't talked much about fruit. Generally speaking, you won't be having fruit on your weight-loss plan because we are trying to minimize the amount of insulin your body releases. But it helps to know how fruit fits into the whole carbohydrate continuum.

Let's look at where fruit fits on the carbohydrate continuum:

ALCOHOL	SUGARS	WHITE THINGS	BROWN THINGS	GREEN THINGS
Grape juice	Raisins Bananas Oranges Apples Peaches Orange juice		Strawberries Blueberries Raspberries	

Seeing where fruit falls on the continuum will help you understand why it will get in the way of your weight-loss plan. However, if you are feeling really cranky one day and want a special treat, you can use fruit to help you through it. Choose one of the slowest fruits (blueberries, strawberries, or raspberries) and have a small bowl with a little bit of cream. The cream will slow the sugar impact down a little, and it also adds a nice flavor. If using cream makes you sad because it's not ice cream, don't use the cream. If using cream makes you want to have more cream immediately, don't have it. Remember, of course, that there is a trade-off for these choices. But use your own judgment as you move into the weight loss process.

Decrease the Amount of Fat You Consume

As you shift into diet mode, you will need to pay attention to your fat levels. I discovered that C57 mice exhibit a disproportionate weight gain and altered body composition in response to a high fat diet.[14] The C57 mice actually gained more weight on high-fat diets without consuming more calories than their normal mouse friends.[20] Researchers found that the genetic differences in metabolic response to fat are more important in the development of obesity and diabetes than the increased caloric content of a high-fat diet.[30] I found this research very comforting because it really helps to explain why we get fat. We are drawn to fat because it evokes beta-endorphin and comforts us. Because of our sugar-sensitive bodies, we gain more weight. We need more comfort. We get fatter even if we are eating less.

Reducing fat from 40 to 30 percent of your total daily intake can have a dramatic effect on your insulin resistance and your capacity to burn rather than store fat. As I started to do the research for this book, I found a journal article titled "Insulin insensitivity is rapidly reversed in rats by reducing dietary fat from 40 to 30% of energy."[31] It got my attention. Let me quote one of its findings: "A moderate reduction in fat intake, from 40 to 30% of energy, can produce a rapid improvement in insulin sensitivity in insulin-insensitive rats, independent of changes in body fat content and irrespective of the means used to reduce dietary fat content." This means that before the rats ever went on a diet, and before they lost any weight, their insulin sensitivity changed dramatically when the fat intake was cut down. Shifting from 40 to 30 percent fat is not a big deal. But it does require a shift in your thinking. For most of the last few years of working with clients, I have encouraged them to use some fat to take the edge off their sugar withdrawal. Consuming fat evokes beta-endorphin. I figured that fat evokes less insulin than sugar, so moderate levels of fat would be a safe alternative to our previously high sugar intake. But I never defined "moderate."

Based on this new research, I am changing my position for those who want to lose weight. You **do** need to pay attention to fat. Use your journal. If your fat level is high, cutting it to below 30 percent of calories will profoundly help your weight loss program. A fat intake of 25 to 28 percent seems to be ideal. Do what you can to bring your fat level down to there. The payoff is worth the commitment.

There is a second intriguing finding about the role of fats in your diet plan. Most of us, including me, have always thought fat was fat. At one point on our website we were discussing the advantage of increasing omega-3 fatty acids for general health purposes. One of our *Your Last Diet!* members reported that she had significantly upped the amount of omega-3 fats she was using and had started losing weight. We were both intrigued, and I went back to the literature to ask whether the *kind* of fat makes a difference. What I found was very exciting. All dietary fats do not increase body fat stores equally.[32]

Bodies eating omega-3 fats rather than things such as beef fat (also called lard) actually burn hotter and consume more energy. Good fats not only increate the heat in your body (thus burning more calories), but reduce the serum triglyceride level.[33] In one study triglyceride levels were *ten times lower* after five weeks of replacing saturated fats with fish oil.[34] That means the fats are being burned rather than floating in your blood.

There is even more. Omega-3 fats actually alter the structure of fat cells. Eating a high-fat diet fills existing fat cells and also stimulates the development of things called adipose precursor cells, or new fat cells in waiting.[35] What contributes to growing fatter is the conversion of these little pre–fat cells into full-blown storage bins. I like to think of it as the storage company planning for the future. They watch how the units are being filled and start framing in new ones, creating a whole row of skeleton units waiting to be finished. The kind of fat you eat decides whether the units will be converted. Bad fats actually speed up the process of converting the precursor cells into active storage units. Good fats—oils containing omega-3 fatty acids (fish and flaxseed oils)—interfere with the conversion. Scientists refer to this as suppressing the late phase

of adipocyte differentiation.[36] Now you can tell your doctor that your salmon dinner is stopping your adipocyte
differentiation.

Not only do omega-3 fatty acids interfere with the conversion of new cells, they seem to affect the actual volume
of existing cells. One study shows that there was a two- to
threefold decrease in fat volume in animals given fish oils.
Even though there was no decrease in the number of fat
cells, the cells emptied out when the animals started to
have fish oil.[37] Think about what this means for you. If you
change the type of fat you are consuming, it will actually
support your weight loss from the inside out.

Diets rich in omega-3 fatty acids seem to increase lipase action.[36] Lipase is responsible for removing fat from
the blood and oxidizing it in the tissues. It may well be
that as we increase our omega-3 fatty acid stores, we are
actually restoring our ability to oxidize fat.

These fascinating animal studies don't rigorously address the implications for human obesity, but shifting
from beef fat to fish fat seems to be a potentially beneficial action without side effects or increased cost. It also
supports your weight loss without damaging your heart
health or contributing to arteriosclerosis. It also avoids
the risk of addiction and withdrawal that comes with the
use of amphetamine-based diet medications.

These studies may also explain why the low-fat craze of
the last ten years has contributed to so many people gaining weight. Low fat means high sugar or increased white
things. Low fat also means low omega-3 fatty acids. Put
these together in a sugar-sensitive body and you will get
weight gain. Fix the sides of the equation and you will
have a successful program.

In sorting out how to create these changes in your fat and fatty acid balance, you need to take a few simple steps. These include:

- Decreasing the amount of saturated fats you eat directly, such as animal fat and butter
- Decreasing the amount of foods you eat that are made with saturated fats such as lard, butter, or margarine
- Increasing your intake of foods that are high in omega-3 fatty acids, such as cold-water fish (salmon, mackerel, sardines, and tuna), or flaxseed and flaxseed oil.

While you are in the process of losing weight, you may want to supplement your intake of omega-3s. You can do this by taking oils that are high in these fatty acids. How much omega-3 oil you take depends on a number of variables, including how fat you are, how much saturated fat you eat, whether you use margarine, and how healthy you are.

A good base dose is to take 1 tablespoon of oil per day if you weigh up to 200 pounds and 2 tablespoons if you weigh more than that. If you have a lot of health problems or if you eat a lot of other fats or margarine, you may want to choose a fish oil higher in omega-3s as a way to get your body more in balance. If you are vegetarian or do not like the way fish oil smells, use flaxseed oil. If you are pregnant or lactating, do not use flaxseed oil.

If you find that you get a fish taste or oil taste when you burp, this may mean you are low in the enzyme lipase. Simply get some digestive enzymes from your local health food store. Read the label to ensure they contain lipase. Do not use them if you have an ulcer or irritable bowel syndrome.

Use this chart to get a sense of how different oils stack up.

OILS	DOSAGE	OMEGA-3	OMEGA-6	RATIO
Flaxseed oil	1 tbsp	6 grams	1.8 grams	3:1 (approx.)
Udo's oil	1 tbsp	6.4 grams	3.2 grams	2:1
Salmon oil	14 capsules	14 grams	0.0 grams	14:0
Essential Balance	1 tbsp	5 grams	5.0 grams	1:1

Many of us simply add 1 tablespoon of omega-3-containing oil to our morning George's shake or use one of these oils on the potato in place of butter. One thing to be very careful about is that these oils are very fragile. Keep them cool, keep them in a dark container, and keep them away from air.

Making small changes can have a big impact on both your health and your weight loss. You do not have to make yourself crazy about this, just add some omega-3s and reduce your overall fat intake.

Planning for Weight Loss

As you plan your weight loss process, pay attention to the demands of your life. Think through what the week will bring. Will you have to catch a 6 A.M. flight on Wednesday? Will you be staying with your brother, who doesn't eat breakfast and has nothing in the house? Will your teenage sons be home and eating everything in sight? Will your spouse or partner be gone for the week? Have you been sick? Will you be working late nights and under a great deal of stress? Breakfast comes every morning. Plan for it.

When you are dieting, it is very easy to skip a meal or start cutting back on the amounts you are eating. A lot of people have written to tell me they are doing the program perfectly and are not losing weight. When I ask them to tell me specifically what they are eating, they send a food journal that outlines very small portions of food. They are in diet mode, and their metabolisms have slowed way down to accommodate less food. When I ask them about this, they always say, "But Kathleen, I feel so much better if I don't eat very much."

There is actually some truth to this observation. As you have already learned, people who are sugar sensitive seem to have lower levels of beta-endorphin. The result is that you unconsciously seek experiences or substances that will help to raise your beta-endorphin level. One of the most intriguing methods you choose is to *not* eat. When you don't eat, your body gets worried. It begins to think you are starving. In its wisdom and kindness, it wants to protect you from the pain of starvation. So it releases a painkiller: beta-endorphin. Got that?

Not eating = Beta-endorphin release

Not eating makes you feel better, more confident, leaner, and more in control because you are getting a beta-endorphin-induced "high." When you cut calories, skip meals, and go for long periods of not eating, your body thinks you are starving. It releases beta-endorphin to numb the pain, and you ride the beta-endorphin wave until you crash. You crash because you go into beta-endorphin withdrawal. When this happens, you eat anything in sight, fall off your food plan, and feel hopeless, out of control, inadequate, and guilty. Do not skip meals, and most especially do not skip breakfast.

Today is day 173 for me. And as of this morning I have dropped seventeen pounds on this plan. The interesting thing about this is that in the beginning I gained and then I had long periods where I lost nothing, then a bit, then nothing. Now that I added exercise to the equation, it seems pretty steady.

It seemed slow, but the bottom line is this—I averaged a pound every ten days. It is steady progress. One hundred seventy-three days is almost six months, and if this were a regular diet I would have lost twenty pounds the first month and the second month gained back thirty, done four more diets, and have ended up in the long run up ten or twenty pounds and disgusted with myself. Instead, I feel radiant, wonderful, successful, well, and hopeful. That in and of itself is enough. The weight loss is a bonus. I don't think I have truly faithfully stuck to any weight loss plan in my life for six months before. There was always cheating and bingeing. This time there is just day-to-day steady. I am so grateful for *Your Last Diet!*

Ruth

Do not create a false beta-endorphin high by cutting down on what you eat. This plan is about abundance, not deprivation. You want to get the perfect amount. And planning is the best way to do this. If you go back and look at Martha's meal planner on p. 60, you will see that there would be very few changes to her food as she starts the diet phase of her plan. She will be eating the same amounts of protein, more vegetables, and slightly fewer brown things. She would stick with a small potato and pay attention to the fats and oils. *Your Last Diet!* is not complex. You know the drill, and you are ready to see a return from all your hard work.

9

The Other Factors
Affecting Weight Loss

If you still have trouble losing weight after doing the
seven steps and the diet, something else may be affecting your ability to lose weight successfully, such as the degree of your insulin resistance, your thyroid function, or
food allergies. Let's take a look at each of these so you can
sort out whether they apply to you.

Insulin Resistance

As you remember, the C57 mice are highly prone to
insulin resistance. Because you are sugar sensitive and
overweight, the chances of your being insulin resistant
are very high. Insulin resistance is a complex subject, and
while there has been a fair amount of discussion about it
in the media during the past few years, few people who
are dieting really understand its implications for weight
loss.

Before I figured out I was sugar sensitive, I heard

about the problem of insulin resistance. Atkins started teaching about it twenty years ago. Ezrin wrote a fascinating book called The *Endocrine Control Diet* in the early nineties. *Protein Power, The Zone, The Carbohydrate Addict's Diet,* and the new, revised Atkins plan have all added to my basic understanding of insulin resistance. But trying to make sense of all that talk of glucose and glycogen and "don't eat carbs" felt overwhelming. I thought, "Ah, just stop eating carbs and you will be fine."

So I would give up all carbs, and I'd feel fabulous, lose weight, and be thrilled. Then, four to six weeks into it, I would get really crabby and really unsettled, and I'd say, "I *have* to have some bread." I would have just a little, and *pow*—I would be on a bread run and then a sugar run, and I'd gain back the weight I lost and more. I would feel hopeless, overwhelmed, ugly, inadequate, and fat. Each time it would get worse and I would be fatter.

Through the personal and professional work that led me to *Potatoes Not Prozac,* I started to make sense of what happened with the *pow.* I learned how beta-endorphin priming and brain upregulation create a bread-induced "drug run." I understood all that and felt absolutely confident that the food plan I had developed would protect against a reenactment of the *pow* effect. But I still couldn't make sense of the insulin resistance story. I needed to revisit this piece and understand what insulin is, what it does, how it is supposed to work, and what contributes to its dysfunction. Let me take you through the sequence that helped me see how the pieces fit together.

Some Background

First of all, let's look at how normal metabolism works. Food provides fuel for the body. Different kinds of food have different functions. Carbohydrates such as sugars, breads, pasta, fruits, and vegetables provide the basic fuel that our bodies burn in order to function. Our muscles, tissues, and brains all use glucose, the simplest sugar, which is derived from carbohydrates.

The carbohydrates are used in three ways: first as fuel for daily life, then as stored energy for later use, and finally as highly concentrated stored energy for the very lean times. The original system evolved in our earliest ancestors, who got lots of exercise and ate food depending upon what time of year it was. During the summer and early fall, carbohydrates such as fruits and vegetables were abundant. People ate more of these foods, stored the excess as fat, and were able to survive the winter, when there was less food available.

Three major changes took place: Food became available all the time, highly refined foods such as sugars and white things became a staple of the diet, and new lifestyles demanded less exercise. The system designed to create fat during the summer and fall as preparation for the lean winter broke down. When our glucose system first evolved, people were not drinking wine or eating bagels or ice cream. Pasta and Halloween candy were not around yet. And people moved a lot. Exercise meant survival; no one hopped in the car to go to McDonald's. So the system worked really well. The change in eating and exercising patterns, however, created a shift in the carbohydrate/insulin/fat-burning balance.

Let's look at this more closely to understand how this shift can affect your body. Carbohydrates are long chains of sugars. During digestion, your body takes the chains apart to make the sugars more and more simple until what remains is glucose, the simplest and most usable form. The longer the chain, the longer it takes to break down. I call the long-chain carbohydrates slow carbs. The length of the chain, the total amount of the carbohydrate eaten, and the amount and type of fat eaten with the carbohydrate all affect absorption rate and blood sugar.

A normal body is set up to function at an optimal level of glucose. It needs to have enough glucose to keep the brain active and to make sure the cells have what they need. The body also needs a storage system to tide it over when the person isn't eating. The body converts the glucose to glycogen and puts it away in the muscles and liver, where it can be easily retrieved later. Glycogen allows the glucose to "keep" longer. I think of it as freeze-dried glucose. Think of the muscles as the kitchen cabinets and the liver as your garage. The extra supplies are put there until needed. But they are close by and it is easy to go get what is necessary. The glycogen in the muscles and liver is meant for short-term needs, like the time between dinner and breakfast—ten hours, not twenty-four.

The third storage place is in the fat cells. Think of these as the storage center down the street. This is where the body puts stuff it doesn't need very often. Fat cells were designed to protect metabolism when times were lean. Fat cells were for winter, when the hunters hadn't found any meat for weeks. Fat cells actually were life-giving in those times. The ones who were fatter were the ones who survived.

The Role of Insulin

Glucose in muscle was really important to early humans—it meant that they had the energy to go out and get more food. Legs walking and running meant staying alive. The hormone called insulin is responsible for getting the glucose in the blood into the cells. The pancreas releases the hormone into the blood, and it swims around looking for insulin receptor sites throughout the body. Insulin goes and tells the cells, "Hey, guys, delivery time. Got what you need. Open up." When the insulin hits the insulin receptor, the cell opens, sucks the glucose into the cell, and says, "Burn, baby." The cell then uses the glucose to make energy. It helps to think of the insulin as a key that turns the lock on the cell door to let the glucose in.

How well the key works in the lock plays a huge part in how you feel and how fat you become. If the key sticks or jams, the cell doesn't open. Or if the key is used over and over and over, it wears down and can't make the connection, so the lock doesn't open and the glucose doesn't get into the cell. You end up with glucose in your blood (high blood sugar) and cells that are starving. You produce insulin, but your cells are resistant to its message. This is called insulin resistance.

Your body is really committed to getting the lock to work. If the first key isn't effective, the body sends another and another. It produces more insulin to try to make the message get through. While the extra insulin sent out may finally get the lock to open, this excess creates more of a problem. What your pancreas thinks is a best solution is actually making it worse. If your cells are bathed in a lot of insulin, they reduce the number of insulin receptors, so there are fewer places where the "burn" message can be recorded. This downregulation—the same thing that happens to beta-endorphin receptors when you eat lots of sugars—means that burning efficiency is reduced. Your insulin resistance increases one more level.

When the system works properly, here is what happens:

- You eat carbohydrates, and they are digested into glucose.
- Insulin is released in proportion to the amount of carbohydrates eaten.
- The insulin message works, and the glucose goes from the blood into the cells to be used for fuel.
- You burn what you need, and there isn't a lot left over.

If you eat more carbohydrates than you actually need to fuel your body, or if you are eating the amount of carbohydrates that you should use but you are insulin resistant and can't use those carbs properly, your body will try to store the extra for later. If your body has filled the cupboards (your muscles) and the shelves in the garage (your liver) with glycogen, the extra needs to be put away somewhere: it goes to the storage unit down the street (your fat stores).

This story seems reasonable, yes? Eat food; store what you don't eat. If you eat too much or eat more than you need, you will get fat, right? Seems to make sense.

Indeed, this theory of what goes in and what goes out is still held by many professionals. They tell you simply to eat less and you will lose weight. They say that for every 3,600 fewer calories you eat, you will lose one pound of body weight.

The Irony for Sugar Sensitives

But this isn't true for many sugar sensitives. How much fat you store does not seem to correlate to how much you eat. Sometimes you eat less than your normal friends do and still gain weight. Sometimes you don't lose weight even if you eat 800 calories a day for three weeks. Many health professionals do not believe this and tell you that if you are fat, it has to be because you eat too much and don't exercise. You *know* that your body works differently, but there has been no validation for your intuition.

Insulin resistance can explain why some people can eat all the carbs they want and gain no weight, while some will seem to gain weight at the sight of an extra carb on the shelf. A genetically inherited tendency to insulin resistance is activated and made worse by what and how you eat. This is especially true if you have a sugar-sensitive biochemistry, because you may produce more insulin than you need.

Insulin resistance becomes even more of a problem if you are overweight. Your fat-to-muscle ratio has a huge impact on how much fuel you need. Muscle cells contain insulin receptors because muscles need glucose as fuel. People with more muscle and leaner muscle need more burning power and have more insulin receptor sites. Fat does not have insulin receptor sites. It just sort of sits there passively, waiting to be called. People with a higher proportion of fat to muscle have fewer insulin receptor sites than people with less fat and more muscle. People with more fat than muscle have way fewer places to burn. People with 44 percent body fat are going to burn a whole lot less than people with 27 percent body fat. You may have intuitively figured this out but didn't understand how the insulin part fit in. So your sense that you can eat the same amount of food as your muscled friend and gain weight while your friend doesn't is on target.

What You Eat Affects Insulin Resistance

Different foods evoke varying degrees of insulin response. As you know from our earlier discussion, scientists have spent a fair amount of time studying how different carbohydrates affect the release of insulin, and many of the recent popular diet programs are designed to address the problem of insulin resistance. "Cut the carbs, increase the protein, and don't worry so much about fat," they say. This strategy does decrease the amount of insulin and will reduce your insulin resistance. This is why these programs have so much appeal. They have a dramatic effect—for *a little while*. But they do not address the role of fats in the insulin story.

A high-fat diet contributes to insulin resistance. How much fat you eat matters in a big way. You may initially lose weight on the high-protein/low-carb diets by reducing your carbohydrates, but the increased fat levels wreak havoc by actually increasing your insulin resistance over time. This effect doesn't show up for a while. While you are rejoicing over your weight loss, your body will be setting the stage for trouble down the line. The first time works, but your body changes, your insulin resistance increases, and the next time you try to use one of these diets, you cannot get the same results.

There is more bad news. Your body needs carbohydrates to function. Carbohydrates provide fuel. They give you energy. Your muscles need them in order to ignite the burn process. Your muscles can use fat as fuel, but the glucose that comes from the carbohydrate serves to ignite the longer-burning fat. Shifting to a high-protein/low-carb diet skews the balance and contributes to metabolic dysfunction.

Protecting Serotonin Levels

In addition, as a sugar-sensitive person, you need to guard your serotonin levels. Effective serotonin function demands a strategic intake of carbohydrates. If you are working rigorously to reduce the carbs without under-standing the effect of the reduction on your brain, you are going to get into trouble. If you are sugar sensitive and have low serotonin, you need a controlled insulin re-sponse to make sure the tryptophan you get from protein can cross over into your brain and make serotonin. If you work really hard to minimize anything that produces an insulin response, you will end up shortchanging your serotonin. And the serotonin is what gives you impulse control. This is part of the reason why after six weeks on the Atkins or Heller plan, your ability to just say no goes out the window and you feel cranky, depressed, and rag-ing for something sweet.

You need to reduce the overall insulin level, but you also want to take care of serotonin as well. Here is where the potato comes in. Yes, it has a high glycemic index score, and yes, it causes a release of insulin. This is exactly what you want: one carefully timed, strategic insulin "hit" for serotonin that will keep your mood up, enhance your impulse control, and stave off depression. The ol' spud works.

The Solutions to Insulin Resistance

So let's review what the steps are in healing your insulin resistance:

1. You want to increase your cells' insulin sensitivity.
2. You want to increase your body's fuel-burning action.
3. You want to maintain your serotonin at optimum levels.

"Yeah, right," you say. Although this whole package seems somewhat daunting, there is good news. Ironically, even though the problem of insulin resistance is incredibly complex, the solution is not. The solution is pretty simple. Not necessarily easy to do, because it does require commitment. But it *is* simple.

Here are the things that you need to do to treat insulin resistance:

- Reduce the amount of insulin-producing foods you eat.
- Maintain an adequate amount of slow carbohydrates.
- Eat a well-timed dose of complex carbohydrates.
- Reduce the amount of fat you eat to 30 percent of your total intake.
- Choose the fats (omega-3s) that enhance fat burning rather than contributing to fat storage.
- Increase your exercise.

The good news is, you are already on the way to doing it! As you do the food plan, stay steady, eat your evening potato, reduce fat (particularly bad fats), and start to exercise, you are treating your insulin resistance.

So what is new about this plan? Why is this any different from what you have been hearing in other diets? Isn't this just one more "cut the calories, cut the fat, cut the carbs, and exercise" plan? Ironically, on one level it is, but on another level, it works in a way that other plans cannot. I am going to show you exactly what part each of these recommendations plays in healing your body so that you never have to diet again. There is no magic here, just solid science and lots of experience. You already know what to do, and I am going to tell you why it will work so well.

Let's go back to the solution steps for healing insulin resistance and really understand the reasoning behind each of my recommendations.

Increase Your Insulin Sensitivity

You want to increase the receptivity of your insulin receptor sites, and you want your body to make more receptors so that the glucose in your blood will get sucked up and burned as fuel. If it is burned, it won't be stored as fat. To increase the number of receptor sites (called upregulation), you need to decrease the amount of insulin produced by your body. You do this by cutting down on the foods that produce insulin—sugar, sweets, and white things. So to decrease your insulin resistance you will reduce eating insulin-producing foods. You have already started this part and made significant gains. What you thought was simply changing whites to browns and going off sugar to get balanced was setting the stage for your weight loss.

Change the Way Your Body Burns Fuel

Having regular and healthy carbs is essential to the function of your brain and body. Highly complex carbs, the brown and green ones—whole grains and vegetables—are slow, so they don't spike your insulin. Shifting from white to brown is not simply about getting you away from the danger foods. It actually goes to the heart of insulin resistance. You have already shifted the proportion of browns and greens as you want to lose weight because vegetables are slower than grains, that is, they have a lower score on the glycemic index. Vegetables will reduce the insulin response the most and will help reduce insulin resistance. As you increase the vegetables, you are helping to increase your insulin sensitivity. At the same time, though, it is critical to keep eating some browns. If the proportion of browns gets too low, you may get cranky and restless. Finding the right combination for you is an art, not a prescription. This is why you have to sort out what is right for you. Use your journal to help your body guide you in finding your own best ratio.

Maintain Your Serotonin Levels

A successful plan will balance competing needs. Yes, you want to decrease the insulin in your system as much as possible. But there is one dilemma. In order to maintain adequate levels of serotonin in your brain and body, you need some insulin to get the amino acid tryptophan into the serotonin factory. Here is the beauty of the potato: It is food as pharmacology. Spuds increase your serotonin in a very contained way. You raise your insulin level at a specific time, using a specific dose for a specific purpose.

Maintaining your serotonin levels is critical to your long-term diet success. Losing weight requires being able to say no to foods as well as patterns of dealing with food. Saying no is the key function of impulse control, which is created by your serotonin levels. Use the potato to increase your serotonin and you will discover a whole new level of self-discipline. The potato, as simple as it is, buys you successful dieting.

The ability to say no is far bigger than saying no to a hot-fudge sundae. It is also the ability to say no to distraction. It means sticking with it, hanging in there, staying at it. We might say it provides the tools for saying yes. Think of your daily spud as giving you the flip side of no—the yes side. Remember to have your evening carb every single day. It counts.

So insulin resistance and your relationship to fats are important factors to consider in designing your weight loss program. There are two other variables to check out as you are refining what you eat: thyroid function and food allergies.

Thyroid Function

If your thyroid gland is not working properly, achieving the right weight loss may be difficult. If your levels of thyroid hormone are low or imbalanced, your metabolism won't heat up and you will not lose weight. At one time I had a tubby, depressed dog with very low thyroid. The vet prescribed medication, and six weeks later she was a different pooch. She lost weight, her coat was sleek and full, and her energy was streaming. Of course, we all yearn for such a magic pill! We hope it will be as simple as our thyroid being off, so we can take pills and get fixed. If you have some of the symptoms of thyroid dysfunction, and especially if you are a woman over forty years old, it is always important to check your thyroid.

Do not assume that thyroid is a magic bullet. Even if your thyroid function is low and you correct it, this may not make a difference in your weight right off the bat. Factor thyroid functioning into your total health picture rather than simply thinking of it as a way to lose weight.

Another Complex Story

The thyroid's functions are confusing, complicated, and contradictory. It can be hard to make informed, clear decisions about your thyroid health without doing some homework. This section will outline the basics for you, but if you want an in-depth, substantive discussion, read Dr. Ridha Arem's *The Thyroid Solution*. It is clear, well written, and expert.

At the most basic level, the thyroid gland produces thyroid hormones that control many of the functions of the body. If the thyroid system isn't working properly and your thyroid levels are low (a condition called hypothyroidism), you can become depressed, gain weight, feel sensitive to cold, have dry skin, and lose hair, to name just a few symptoms. If your thyroid gland is producing too much thyroid (hyperthyroidism), you can be anxious, hyperactive, and exhausted. If you have any of the symptoms listed below and have not had your thyroid checked, you should do so.

First of all, go through this list of the symptoms of low thyroid function and see if they fit your profile:

- Weight gain disproportionate to diet
- Depression
- Dry hair or skin
- Hair loss
- Increased menstrual flow
- Puffiness
- Brittle nails
- Cold intolerance
- Fatigue
- Constipation
- Dry eyes
- Shortness of breath when exercising

The two symptoms affecting most sugar sensitives are weight gain and depression. You can be doing everything right and still not be losing weight. If you are working a diligent, committed program, still aren't losing weight, and still feel dark and sad, then it's time for a thyroid check.

If you have all the symptoms of low thyroid and in your gut you believe that you are hypothyroid but you are told that the lab values are normal, this can be frustrating. Often the lab report is given with one more medical message of "If you would just exercise or stop eating so much, you could lose the weight." Without understanding how the thyroid works or how normal lab values are constructed, this message can be intimidating, particularly if you are at an early stage in your recovery. If you have your thyroid tested after you are stable and free of mush brain, you can simply be proactive in sorting out what is going on, and understanding how the lab works can help. Lab measurements show a dysfunctional or normal thyroid within certain parameters set by a given lab. But there is such a thing as subclinical thyroid disease, in which lab values fall at the extremes of what some clinicians consider normal, and you need a doctor who understands this. Arem talks about the need to know what is normal for you versus what is normal for most of the population.

How the Thyroid Works

Let's take a look at how the thyroid system works, where things can go wrong, and how to work with your doctor to discover if thyroid function is a part of your problem. Now, I don't have all the answers for you and am not an expert on the thyroid, but I can help you ask the right questions and show you how to see the pieces more easily. Here are the players in the thyroid system:

TRH is thyroid-releasing hormone. It is made in the hypothalamus and acts on the pituitary gland to change the levels of TSH.

TSH is thyroid-stimulating hormone. The pituitary gland senses how much thyroid is circulating in the blood and reacts to any change by adjusting the TSH production. The level of TSH instructs the thyroid gland to make more or less thyroid hormone. The TSH and the thyroid create a feedback loop to maintain the amount of thyroid hormone at an optimal level.

Your level of TSH goes up if your thyroid gland is producing too little thyroid hormone. An elevated level of TSH says your thyroid production is low. The level of TSH is a highly reliable measure of your thyroid function.

Because the thyroid gland needs iodine, selenium, and zinc to do its job, it is important to ensure that you have optimal levels of these in your diet.

T4 and **T3** are the two actual hormones made by the thyroid gland. Thyroid hormones are made when the gland combines molecules of iodine with molecules of the amino acid tyrosine. You need to have the iodine and the amino acid for your thyroid gland to be able to manufacture the hormones properly. If you live in an area where there is little iodine available, or if you eat few foods that contain iodine, your thyroid will struggle to make the hormone. When it struggles for a long time, the gland gets bigger, a condition called goiter, and you may even experience low-grade hypothyroidism.

Your body converts T4 to T3 by the action of a specific enzyme. Usually your body will have thirty times more T4 than T3, but it is the T3 that acts most dramatically at the cellular level. If the conversion enzyme doesn't work properly, your body won't convert T4 to T3 the way it needs to. Or your body may convert the T4 to something called reverse T3, which does not do the job. Some researchers believe that toxins may interfere with the conversion process. You may have enough T4 but not have the proper amount of T3.

T3 regulates what is called thermogenesis, or oxygen-associated burning at the cellular level. Without adequate T3, the cells don't work properly, and your body won't create the heat that burns fat.

Receptor Functioning

Thyroid hormone works by attaching to a receptor site (very much the way the neurotransmitters beta-endorphin and serotonin attach to receptors that are specific to them). When the thyroid hormone activates the thyroid receptors, its regulating message is sent to the cells. You may be producing adequate T4, and you may be converting T4 to T3 properly, but if the hormone can't get into the cell to do its job, the net effect will be low thyroid action. There are some drugs, such as beta-blockers, that interfere with the hormone action.

There are also some foods that interfere with thyroid function, including cabbage, Brussels sprouts, turnips, and broccoli. Now, this does not mean you should avoid these foods. But if you are eating huge amounts of these uncooked (or raw) vegetables, and have symptoms of low thyroid, be aware of this effect and factor it in as you sort out how to get better.

Let's go back over the main points of thyroid function and review all the pieces that need to work properly. You need certain raw materials, including vitamins, minerals, and amino acids, to manufacture thyroid hormone. These include tyrosine (from protein foods), iodine, zinc, selenium, and vitamin A. The TSH feedback loop must work properly, and T4 needs to be converted to T3 properly. The T3 needs to bind to the receptor sites properly.

Now, of course, you can't know all these pieces specifically. But you can be informed about the different pieces and learn to understand what your lab values actually are saying.

What to Do?

If you have the symptoms of low thyroid, ask your doctor to order a thyroid panel, which includes your level of TSH. Read Arem's book carefully, particularly the chapter that describes how to interpret lab values.

Because the thyroid hormone regulates metabolism, some doctors and alternative health care practitioners believe that your body temperature can be an indication of low levels of thyroid function. There is disagreement about the usefulness of the basal temperature in measuring thyroid function. It is not absolute, and by itself it is an incomplete measure, but it can add to the total profile you are putting together. If your basal temperature is under 97 degrees, it is possible that your thyroid is not working properly. It is also possible that your thyroid function is fine and you simply are not getting enough exercise to stimulate your metabolism, or you may be suffering from depression.

As you attempt to sort this out, you may find yourself in an interesting position with your doctor. He or she may tell you that your TSH levels are normal and to stop worrying about it. Or on the other end of the scale, some doctors may only have you measure your basal temperature, find that it is low, and then prescribe thyroid supplementation without any further diagnostic tests. This is an incomplete diagnosis and treatment. If you have the symptoms, get the complete picture. Keep working at it until you really understand the pieces and how they fit

together. Reread Arem's book with the ol' yellow highlighter in hand, take notes, and be in charge of your
health.

Food Allergies

Many people have asked me about whether food allergies
play a part in their weight or in cravings. The answer can
be yes to both of these. However, I do not recommend
that you add the allergy piece to your weight loss equation
until *after* your foundation plan is steady and you have
worked your program for a while. Learning that you are
allergic to wheat or dairy can create a sense of panic if
you're at an early stage in your program. Your untreated
sugar-sensitive self would have been hysterical at the idea
of taking out not only sugar but also wheat and dairy.
Your brain could not imagine what would be left to eat
and would tell you to drop this program as quickly as possible. Because of this, I downplay the allergy research until you have the stability to look at it dispassionately.

Sometimes simply doing the program quiets a body
that is reacting allergically. Taking out the sugars, shifting
the types of fats, stabilizing the blood sugar, and creating
a predictable routine may resolve hypersensitivity, so taking out any foods really isn't necessary. On the other
hand, for some sugar sensitives, wheat and dairy allergy
can create havoc in an otherwise stable program. You may
be working a very diligent program and still experience a
"food coma" after lunch, when you can hardly keep your
eyes open. Headaches, bloating, sinus congestion, water
retention, stomach pain, joint pain, and depression can
all come from food allergies. If you have any of these

symptoms after you have been doing the program for a while, it is worth exploring food allergies.

The other big clue, the one I find the most intriguing, is the intensity of your attachment to a given food. If a certain food holds a big emotional attachment, it may be a food you are allergic to. If you eat a food that you are allergic to, your body will produce beta-endorphin to protect you from the stress of the allergic reaction. If you are sugar sensitive, this beta-endorphin release will actually make you feel good. Your brain associates the beta-endorphin euphoria with the particular food, and so you are drawn to the foods that create the allergy. If you love whole wheat bread, milk, or popcorn, for example, you may be getting an allergy-induced high from it.

This reaction can provide a wonderful clue about the potential for food allergy. Use your food journal to see if there is any type of food to which you are particularly drawn. Don't scare yourself about having to give it up. Just start the detective work. It isn't necessary for you to go and get all sorts of expensive tests to work with this. Simply try taking that one food out of your diet and see what happens. Do you start having an anxiety attack even when you simply think about taking it out? Do you get restless and sad? These are clues. If you try to stop using that food, do you get irritable and cranky and start roaming around the house thinking about it? If you try to do this while you are still using sweets and white things, it will be hard to tell whether you are having a hard time with the sugar aspect or the food aspect.

Sometimes people find it almost impossible to give up white things and not so hard to deal with giving up sugar. This can be a function of being allergic to wheat. Wheat, corn, and dairy are the three biggest allergens I see in my clients and readers. You might want to get a copy of *The False Fat Diet* by Elson Haas, M.D. It is one of the best discussions of food allergies I have seen. Dr. Haas is very specific and helpful in getting a sense of what may be going on with food allergies. But do not try to add this piece of the equation into your healing plan until after you are steady with your program.

10

Finding Radiance

I recently got an email from a reader who said, "Kathleen, I have been doing this plan for six weeks. When am I going to get radiant?" It made me laugh. You don't get radiant all at once. You don't get radiant in a few weeks. Radiance doesn't happen in a moment. It will creep up on you in small increments. You will live into it, one choice, one day, one slip, one insight at a time.

In this chapter I am going to talk about things that are not usually part of a diet book. I am going to rewrite the rules to honor the miracle of what you are doing here. Usually, the last chapter is kind of an afterthought. But in *Your Last Diet!* this chapter is really about the promise, the best of what is to come with your plan. This chapter is really the beginning of where you are going. When you got *Your Last Diet!* you figured it would offer you a way to get to your goal weight. I fooled you. It is really about never, ever being caught in that craziness again.

Your first clue will be when you notice that what the

scale says no longer is the most important issue in your life. How you feel will start to emerge as your marker for improvement. Instead of feeling out of control, you will understand *why* you feel the way you do, and you will have an enormous sense of personal power. This shift at a molecular level is the start of living in radiance.

This program brings major, major blessings, doesn't it? Sometimes when I look at my life before *Your Last Diet!* it is simply unfathomable—I know we lived it, but it just doesn't seem like we could have for all those years. Asking us to go back to that life now would be like asking me to hide away from the sun and burrow into a hole in the ground and stay there. Every day was such a struggle, and now, well, now every day is a new adventure. Remember the old axiom "Every day in every way I am getting better and better"? Well, now it's really true! We can add happier and happier, healthier and healthier, stronger and stronger, more and more radiant.

Ruth

What causes this shift that sugar sensitives experience in their healing? It is not just in your head. It isn't simply a change in attitude. It is biochemical—it is in your brain, your blood, your heart, your fingers, and your toes. Your arms feel different. You feel lighter. You are more "there." You have changed the levels of glucose in your blood, you have changed your serotonin levels, and you have changed your beta-endorphin levels. No wonder you feel different.

The shift is everywhere. Do you remember when you

felt depressed and experienced it in your entire body?
You felt as if you could not move your arm, or you simply
could not pick up your leg to go up the stairs. Or you felt
dark all over your body. If serotonin creates a sense of
brightness in your mood, when you have low serotonin
you will feel darkness wherever there was a serotonin
deficit. Serotonin is in platelets and you felt dark wherever you have blood. The world felt dark. It felt all pervasive. But think about this—if it was happening in your
blood cells, it *was* all pervasive. Your blood cells were dark.

Think about having a heavy heart, feeling as if your
heart is dark, grieving, or experiencing trauma or intense
stress. In these situations, your serotonin levels get de-
pleted. But you have different heart feelings when your
serotonin levels are up. Your heart feels light and full.

Do not be surprised about what changes for you. Your
body will change. Your emotions will change. The big feelings, the ones you have struggled with for so long (or the
ones you have buried so deep), will come to you in a way
that is manageable. You will be able to heal them as never
before. You will be able to hold them, understand them,
and share them with people who are safe and supportive.
If you are now in therapy, the quality of your therapy will
change. It will go deeper, become richer. It may become
more painful, but the miracle is that you will be able to
hold whatever comes up and work it through, thanks to
your now stable and strong biochemistry.

If you feel disconnected, either from your family or
from a sense of purpose, this will change as well. The letters that have poured into the www.radiantrecovery.com
website reveal a number of startlingly similar themes. After people had done the program for a while, they moved
though an intriguing developmental process. First they

described a sense of mastery and clarity. They felt at peace and focused. They felt able to manage life. And even if the food got a little wobbly, they knew what to do and how to get back on track.

After a year or so on the program, something very un-expected started to happen. People spontaneously started talking about connection, purpose, and relationship, both to the people they loved and to the divine. I was floored. These discussions were totally outside what we had contracted for. But they spontaneously came, over and over.

> I'm just not sure what this would do to people who haven't started recovery yet. If I had read this book one and a half years ago, I would have thought, "What a load of bullshit"— and it would probably have put me off from buying the book. This is probably the most important of all chapters . . . that's my view now! Radiance is a sense of purpose, connectedness to the "big picture," a feeling of being guided, and the feeling that one glimpse, one little spark is all you need, and the voyage you embark on is beyond anything you were able to imagine before.
>
> *Simone*

How this manifested was different for everyone. Some people were devout Christians who experienced a better relationship with God; some were Twelve-Steppers who reaffirmed the role of their higher power; and some de-fined the divine simply as a feeling of purpose and inten-tion at work in their lives. Whatever they called it, the people who did the steps diligently over time reported a similar experience: deep connection and healing.

Nothing else in their lives had really changed to account for it—nothing except their food. Not one had had a conversion experience; not one came right out and said he or she had had a spiritual awakening. Their lives simply changed. They felt settled, clear, and somehow guided. Things had just shifted, and having a spiritual connection seemed like the natural next step.

What they described was the same journey I had experienced. Do the food and your life will change. Do the food, add in the other pieces that teach you about yourself, and radiance will creep in unbidden. As more and more people described this, I realized that what I had experienced was not simply my own personal experience. It was a function of the program. When you change the food, other things change as well.

Now, sometimes these changes may be hard. Your family and friends may not like the person you are becoming. They may try to sabotage you by offering you desserts, saying, "Just a little sweet won't hurt you." They may accuse you of being fanatic about this fad diet thing; if you get involved with the online community, they may tell you it is a cult and you will get swept away. Your emerging radiance may scare them and make them unsettled. They may feel as if you are judging them for being stuck or caught in old patterns. And sometimes, rather than explore with you, they attack.

Doing the food creates a steady bowl to hold these experiences. As it fills, the connection deepens both inside and outside. You are not afraid; you are not alone. You are part of a larger miracle. You share this understanding with thousands and thousands of sugar-sensitive people all over the world who are making this same change. And through the wonderful technology of the Internet, you can connect directly with this collection of people discovering radiance together. It doesn't matter if you live in Topeka, Seattle, Auckland, Edinburgh, Albuquerque, Portland, Dublin, Singapore, or Cincinnati. You can come home to a community that understands and supports your journey.

You thought that the details of your life were idiosyncratic and personal. You thought you were the only one who struggled with clutter, who loved office supply stores. We felt that, too. We assumed that the shift we felt was simply a personal manifestation of getting better. Then we started sharing and discovered that it is not a personal journey. We felt connected to something big and powerful. We, who had felt disconnected, hopeless, and isolated, now felt ourselves a part of a healing community.

One day at a seminar at Ghost Ranch, we were talking about the role of beta-endorphin in creating a sense of connection and well being. And there at Ghost Ranch we felt really, really connected not only to one another but also to something big! We were talking about the power of beta-endorphin, and we spontaneously said, "This feels like AlphaEndorphin!" Using a new word bridged the old "god" vocabulary, where we got stuck in trying to talk with one another.

We saw that the connection can be to God, Spirit, Father, Mother, Lord, Krishna, or the universe humming. It no longer mattered. The term "AlphaE" created the bridge to describe a shared experience. When we do the food, we feel connected not only to one another, but to AlphaE. It feels as if there is a plan, a meaning, a purpose.

And if the food slips, the connection slides. We forget. We think the sugar feelings are real. We lose a sense of purpose; "radiance" sounds like some stupid marketing catchword; we think, "This dumb diet doesn't work." And we do the food, and radiance starts to breathe us once again.

As you do the food plan, you are going to get more than weight loss. This will be *Your Last Diet!* because the cause of all that turmoil for all those years will be healed. Your sugar feelings will naturally and organically shift. You don't have to work them out. You don't have to work through your self-esteem and take care of fixing your whole life. You just do the food and the feelings will take care of themselves. This is not to say that doing the food will fix everything. Doing the food will balance you, and you will then know exactly what else you need to do to heal yourself.

We are reshaping the story of being fat in a totally new way. *Your Last Diet!* is a living book. We are talking about something way bigger than changing how much you weigh. We are talking about claiming your birthright—the birthright of radiance. I will talk about this more in my next books. You do the food, and together we will write the next chapter of the story.

Notes

1. Goas, J., *Endocrine factors underlying the ethanol preference of C57B1/6j Mice.* Federal proceedings, 1978. 37: p. 421.
2. Surwit, R. S., et al., *Control of expression of insulin resistance and hyperglycemia by different genetic factors in diabetic C57BL/6J mice.* Diabetes, 1991. 40(1): pp. 82–87.
3. Wurtman, R. J., and J. J. Wurtman, *Brain serotonin, carbohydrate-craving, obesity and depression.* Obes Res, 1995. 3(Suppl 4): pp. 477S–480S.
4. Wurtman, J. J., *Carbohydrate craving. Relationship between carbohydrate intake and disorders of mood.* Drugs, 1990. 39(Suppl 3): pp. 49–52.
5. Lowinson, P. R., and R. Millman, *Substance Abuse: A Comprehensive Textbook.* 1992, Baltimore: Williams & Wilkins.
6. Gianoulakis, C., J. P. de Waele, and J. Thavundayil, *Implication of the endogenous opioid system in excessive ethanol consumption.* Alcohol, 1996. 13(1): pp. 19–23.
7. Blass, E., *Opioids, sweets and a mechanism for positive affect: broad motivational implications,* Sweetness, 1987. pp. 115–26.
8. DesMaisons, K., *Biochemical restoration as an intervention for multiple offense drunk driving.* 1996, Cincinnati, OH: The Union Institute.
9. Gianoulakis, C., and J. P. de Waele, *Genetics of alcoholism: role of the endogenous opioid system.* Metab Brain Dis, 1994. 9(2): pp. 105–31.
10. Stewart, R., *Consumption of sweet, salty, sour, and bitter solutions by selectively bred alcohol-preferring and alcohol-nonpreferring lines of rats.* Alcoholism: Clinical and Experimental Research, 1994. 18(2): pp. 375–81.
11. De Waele, J. P., D. N. Papachristou, and C. Gianoulakis, *The alcohol-preferring C57BL/6 mice present an enhanced sensitivity of the hypothala-*

mic beta-endorphin system to ethanol than the alcohol-avoiding DBA/2 mice. J Pharmacol Exp Ther, 1992. 261(2): pp. 788–94.

12. Blass, E., E. Fitzerald, and P. Kehoe, *Interactions between sucrose, pain and isolation distress.* Pharmacol Biochem Behav, 1987. 26(3): pp. 483–89.

13. Tejedor-Real, P., et al., *Involvement of delta-opioid receptors in the effects induced by endogenous enkephalins on learned helplessness model.* Eur J Pharmacol, 1998. 354(1): pp. 1–7.

14. Black, B. L., et al., *Differential effects of fat and sucrose on body composition in A/J and C57BL/6 mice.* Metabolism, 1998. 47(11): pp. 1354–9.

15. Wencel, H. E., et al., *Impaired second phase insulin response of diabetes-prone C57BL/6J mouse islets.* Physiol Behav, 1995. 57(6): pp. 1215–20.

16. Lee, S. K., et al., *Defective glucose-stimulated insulin release from perifused islets of C57BL/6J mice.* Pancreas, 1995. 11(2): pp. 206–11.

17. Parekh, P. I., et al., *Reversal of diet-induced obesity and diabetes in C57BL/6J mice.* Metabolism, 1998. 47(9): pp. 1089–96.

18. Hill, J. O., et al., *Lipid accumulation and body fat distribution is influenced by type of dietary fat fed to rats.* Int J Obes Relat Metab Disord, 1993. 17(4): pp. 223–36.

19. Surwit, R. S., et al., *Differential glycemic effects of morphine in diabetic and normal mice.* Metabolism, 1989. 38(3): pp. 282–85.

20. Surwit, R. S., et al., *Metabolic and behavioral effects of a high-sucrose diet during weight loss.* Am J Clin Nutr, 1997. 65(4): pp. 908–15.

21. Brownlow, B. S., et al., *The role of motor activity in diet-induced obesity in C57BL/6J mice.* Physiol Behav, 1996. 60(1): pp. 37–41.

22. Pennington, J., *Food Values of Portions Commonly Used.* 1994, Philadelphia: J. B. Lippincott Co.

23. Jenkins, D. J., et al., *Glycemic index of foods: a physiological basis for carbohydrate exchange.* Am J Clin Nutr, 1981. 34(3): pp. 362–66.

24. DeAngelis, L. D. K., G. Gadonski, J. Fang, P. Dall'Ago, V. L. Albuquerque, L. R. Peixoto, T. G Fernandes, and M. C. Irigoyen, *Exercise reverses peripheral insulin resistance in trained L-NAME-hypertensive rats.* Hypertension, 1999. 34(4, pt. 2): pp. 768–72.

25. Arciero, P. J., M. D. Vukovich, J. O. Holloszy, S. B. Racette, and W. M. Kohrt, *Comparison of short-term diet and exercise on insulin action in individuals with abnormal glucose tolerance.* J Appl Physiol, 1999. 86(6): pp. 1930–5.

26. Simoneau, J. A., J. H. Veerkamp, L. P. Turcotte, and D. E. Kelley, *Markers of capacity to utilize fatty acids in human skeletal muscle: relation to insulin resistance and obesity and effects of weight loss.* FASEB J, 1999. 13(14): pp. 2051–60.

27. Etgen, G. J. Jr., et al., *Exercise training reverses insulin resistance in muscle by enhanced recruitment of GLUT-4 to the cell surface.* Am J Physiol, 1997. 272(5 Pt 1): pp. E864–69.

28. Schwarz, L., and W. Kindermann, *Changes in beta-endorphin levels in response to aerobic and anaerobic exercise.* Sports Med, 1992. 13(1): pp. 25–36.

29. Kraemer, R. R., et al., *Effects of treadmill running on plasma beta-endorphin, corticotropin, and cortisol levels in male and female 10K runners.* Eur J Appl Physiol Occup Physiol, 1989. 58(8): pp. 845–51.

30. Surwit, R. S., et al., *Diet-induced changes in uncoupling proteins in obesity-prone and obesity-resistant strains of mice.* Proc Natl Acad Sci USA, 1998. 95(7): pp. 4061–5.

31. Harris, R. B., and H. Kor, *Insulin insensitivity is rapidly reversed in rats by reducing dietary fat from 40 to 30% of energy.* J Nutr, 1992. 122(9): pp. 1811–22.

32. Bell, R. R., M. J. Spencer, and J. L. Sheriff, *Voluntary exercise and monounsaturated canola oil reduce fat gain in mice fed diets high in fat.* J Nutr, 1997. 127(10): pp. 2006–10.

33. Shimomura, Y., T. Tamura, and M. Suzuki, *Less body fat accumulation in rats fed a safflower oil diet than in rats fed a beef tallow diet.* J Nutr, 1990. 120(11): pp. 1291–6.

34. Parrish, C. C., et al., *Dietary fish oils modify adipocyte structure and function.* J Cell Physiol, 1991. 148(3): pp. 493–502.

35. Klyde, B. J., and J. Hirsch, *Increased cellular proliferation in adipose tissue of adult rats fed a high-fat diet.* J Lipid Res, 1979. 20(6): pp. 705–15.

36. Okuno, M., et al., *Perilla oil prevents the excessive growth of visceral adipose tissue in rats by down-regulating adipocyte differentation.* J Nutr, 1997. 127(9): pp. 1752–7.

37. Parrish, C. C., D. A. Pathy, and A. Angel, *Dietary fish oils limit adipose tissue hypertrophy in rats.* Metabolism, 1990. 39(3): pp. 217–9.

Bibliography

Abrahamson, E. M., and A. W. Pezet, *Body, Mind and Sugar.*. 1951, New York, NY: Henry Holt and Company.

Adamec, R., *Transmitter systems involved in neural plasticity underlying increased anxiety and defense—implications for understanding anxiety following traumatic stress.* Neurosci Biobehav Rev, 1997. 21(6): pp. 755–65.

Agren, J. J., et al., *Fish diet, fish oil and docosahexaenoic acid rich oil lower fasting and postprandial plasma lipid levels.* Eur J Clin Nutr, 1996. 50(11): pp. 765–71.

Alberici, J. C., et al., *Effects of preexercise candy bar ingestion on glycemic response, substrate utilization, and performance.* Int J Sport Nutr, 1993. 3(3): pp. 323–33.

Anderson, I. M., et al., *Dieting reduces plasma tryptophan and alters brain 5-HT function in women.* Psychol Med, 1990. 20(4): pp. 785–791.

Arciero, P. J., et al., *Comparison of short-term diet and exercise on insulin action in individuals with abnormal glucose tolerance.* J Appl Physiol, 1999. 86(6): pp. 1930–5.

Bartness, T. J., et al., *Reversal of high-fat diet-induced obesity in female rats.* Am J Physiol, 1992. 263(4 Pt 2): pp. R790–97.

Behall, K. M., D. J. Scholfield, and J. Hallfrisch, *Effect of beta-glucan level in oat fiber extracts on blood lipids in men and women.* J Am Coll Nutr, 1997. 16(1): pp. 46–51.

Behme, M. T., *Dietary fish oil enhances insulin sensitivity in miniature pigs.* J Nutr, 1996. 126(6): pp. 1549–53.

Bell, R. R., M. J. Spencer, and J. L. Sheriff, *Voluntary exercise and monosaturated canola oil reduce fat gain in mice fed diets high in fat.* J Nutr, 1997. 127(10): pp. 2006–10.

Bernardis, L. L., and L. L. Bellinger, *Brown (BAT) and white (WAT) adipose tissue in high-fat junk food (HFJF) and chow-fed rats with dorsomedial hypothalamic lesions (DMNL rats).* Behav Brain Res, 1991. 43(2): pp. 191–95.

Bertiere, M. C., et al., *Stress and sucrose hyperphagia: role of endogenous opiates.* Pharmacol Biochem Behav, 1984. 20(5): pp. 675–9.

Bertrand, E., et al., *Social interaction increases the extracellular levels of [Met]enkephalin in the nucleus accumbens of control but not of chronic mild stressed rats.* Neuroscience, 1997. 80(1): pp. 17–20.

Besson, A., et al., *Effects of morphine, naloxone and their interaction in the learned-helplessness paradigm in rats.* Psychopharmacology (Berl), 1996. 123(1): pp. 71–78.

Black, B. L., et al., *Differential effects of fat and sucrose on body composition in A/J and C57BL/6 mice.* Metabolism, 1998. 47(11): pp. 1354–9.

Blair, S., *Evidence for success of exercise in weight loss and control.* Ann Intern Med, 1993. 119(Oct 1): pp. 702–6.

Blass, E., E. Fitzgerald, and P. Kehoe, *Interactions between sucrose, pain and isolation distress.* Pharmacol Biochem Behav, 1987. 26(3): pp. 483–9.

Blass, E. M., *Pain-reducing properties of sucrose in human newborns.* Chem Senses, 1995. 20(1): pp. 29–35.

Bouix, O., et al., *Endogenous oploid peptides stimulate post-exercise insulin response to glucose in rats.* Int J Sports Med, 1996. 17(2): pp. 80–84.

Bourre, J. M., et al., *High dietary fish oil alters the brain polyunsaturated fatty acid composition.* Biochim Biophys Acta, 1988. 960(3): pp. 458–61.

Brown G. L., M.D., *CSF serotonin metabolite (5-HIAA) studies in depression, impulsivity, and violence.* Journal of Clinical Psychiatry, 1990. 51(4): pp. 31–41.

Brown, R., *An Introduction to Neuroendocrinology.* 1994, Cambridge, England: Cambridge University Press.

Brownlow, B. S., et al., *The role of motor activity in diet-induced obesity in C57BL/6J mice.* Physiol Behav, 1996. 60(1): pp. 37–41.

Bujatti, M. P., *Serotonin, noradrenaline, dopamine metabolites in transcendental meditation-technique.* Journal of Neural Transmission, 1976. 39: pp. 257–67.

Caldarone, B. J., et al., *Gender differences in learned helplessness behavior are influenced by genetic background.* Pharmacol Biochem Behav, 2000. 66(4): pp. 811–17.

Carlotti, M., et al., *Beneficial effects of a fish oil enriched high lard diet on obesity and hyperlipemia in Zucker rats.* Ann NY Acad Sci, 1993. 683: pp. 349–50.

Chicco, A., et al., *Effect of moderate levels of dietary fish oil on insulin secre-*

tion and sensitivity, and pancreas insulin content in normal rats. Ann Nutr Metab, 1996. 40(2): pp. 61–70.

Cleary, J., et al., *Naloxone effects on sucrose-motivated behavior.* Psychopharmacology (Berl), 1996. 126(2): pp. 110–14.

Collins, S., et al., *Role of leptin in fat regulation.* Nature, 1996. 380(6576): p. 677.

Cowen, P. J., et al., *Moderate dieting causes 5-HT2C receptor supersensitivity.* Psychol Med, 1996. 26(6): pp. 1155–9.

Czirr, S. A., and L. D. Reid, *Demonstrating morphine's potentiating effects on sucrose-intake.* Brain Research Bulletin, 1986. 17: pp. 639–42.

DeAngelis, L. D. K., G. Gadonski, J. Fang, P. Dall'Ago, V. L. Albuquerque, L. R. Peixoto, T. G. Fernandes, and M. C. Irigoyen. *Exercise reverses peripheral insulin resistance in trained L-NAME-hypertensive rats.* Hypertension, 1999. 34(4 pt. 2): pp. 768–72.

de Waele, J. P., and C. Gianoulakis, *Characterization of the mu and delta opioid receptors in the brain of the C57BL/6J and DBA/2 mice, selected for their differences in voluntary ethanol consumption.* Alcohol Clin Exp Res, 1997. 21(4): pp. 754–62.

de Waele, J. P., K. Kiianmaa, and C. Gianoulakis, *Distribution of the mu and delta opioid binding sites in the brain of the alcohol-preferring AA and alcohol-avoiding ANA lines of rats.* J Pharmacol Exp Ther, 1995. 275(1): pp. 518–27.

De Waele, J. P., D. N. Papachristou, and C. Gianoulakis, *The alcohol-preferring C57BL/6 mice present an enhanced sensitivity of the hypothalamic beta-endorphin system to ethanol than the alcohol-avoiding DBA/2 mice.* J Pharmacol Exp Ther, 1992. 261(2): pp. 788–94.

DeLany, J. P., et al., *Conjugated linoleic acid rapidly reduces body fat content in mice without affecting energy intake.* Am J Physiol, 1999. 276(4 Pt 2); pp. R1172–9.

DesMaisons, K., Biochemical restoration as an intervention for multiple offense drunk driving. 1996, Cincinnati, OH; The Union Institute.

Dess, N. K, *Responses to basic taste qualities in rats selectively bred for high versus low saccharin intake.* Physiol Behav, 2000. 69(3): pp. 247–57.

Doucet, E., et al., *Changes in energy expenditure and substrate oxidation resulting from weight loss in obese men and women: is there an important contribution of leptin?* J Clin Endocrinol Metab, 2000. 85(4): pp. 1550–6.

Dragon, N., et al., *Primary structure and morphine-like activity of human beta-endorphin.* Can J Biochem, 1977. 55(6): pp. 666–70.

Drewnowski, A., et al., *Naloxone, an opiate blocker, reduces the consumption of sweet high-fat foods in obese and lean female binge eaters.* Am J Clin Nutr, 1995. 61(6): pp. 1206–12.

Drewnowski, A., S. A. Henderson, and A. Barratt-Fornell, *Genetic sensitivity to 6-n-propylthiouracil and sensory responses to sugar and fat mixtures.* Physiol Behav, 1998. 63(5): pp. 771–7.

Drewnowski, A., S. A. Henderson, and A. Barratt–Fornell, *Genetic taste markers and food preferences.* Drug Metab Dispos, 20021. 29(4 Pt 2): pp. 535–8.

Drewnowski, A. and M. Schwartz, *Invisible fats: sensory assessment of sugar/fat mixtures.* Appetite, 1990. 14(3): pp. 203–17.

Eipper, B. A., and R. E. Mains, *The role of ascorbate in the biosynthesis of neuroendocrine peptides.* Am J of Clin Nutr, 1991. 54: pp. 1153s–1156s.

Esposito-Del Puente, A., et al., *Glycemic response to stress is altered in euglycemic Pima Indians.* Int J Obes Relat Metab Disord, 1994. 18(11): pp. 766–70.

Etgen, G. J., Jr., et al., *Exercise training reverses insulin resistance in muscle by enhanced recruitment of GLUT-4 to the cell surface.* Am J Physiol, 1997. 272(5 Pt 1): pp. E864–69.

Everly, G. S., Jr., *Psychotraumatology: a two-factor formulation of post-traumatic stress.* Integr Physio Behav Sci, 1993. 28(3): pp. 270–78.

Fantino, M., J. Hosotte, and M. Apfelbaum, *An opioid antagonist, naltrexone, reduces preference for sucrose in humans.* Am J Physiol, 1986. 251(1 Pt 2): pp. R91–96.

Farrell, P. A., et al., *Beta-endorphin and adrenocorticotropin response to supramaximal treadmill exercise in trained and untrained males.* Acta Physiol Scand, 1987. 130(4): pp. 619–25.

Fedele, F., et al., *Role of the central endogenous opiate system in patients with syndrome X.* Am Heart J, 1998. 136(6): pp. 1003–9.

Fernstrom, J. D., *Effects of precursors on brain neurotransmitter synthesis and brain functions.* Diabetologia, 1981. 20 Suppl: pp. 281–89.

Fernstrom, J. D., and D. V. Faller, *Neutral amino acids in the brain: changes in response to food ingestion.* J Neurochem, 1978. 30(6): pp. 1531–8.

Fernstrom, J. D., and R. J. Wurtman, *Brain serotonin content: increase following ingestion of carbohydrate diet.* Science, 1971, 174(13): pp. 1023–5.

Fernstrom, J. D., and R. J. Wurtman, *Brain serotonin content: physiological regulation by plasma neutral amino acids.* Science, 1972. 178(59): pp. 414–16.

Forsander, O., *Is carbohydrate metabolism genetically related to alcohol drinking?* Alcohol and Alcoholism, 1987. 1: pp. 357–59.

Fremont, L., M. T. Gozzelino, and T. Hojjat, *Effects of moderate fat intake with different n-3 fatty acid sources and n-6/n-3 ratios on serum and structural lipids in rats.* Reprod Nutr Dev, 1995. 35(5): pp. 503–15.

Fullerton, D. T., et al., *Sugar, opioids and binge eating.* Brain Res Bull, 1985. 14(6); pp. 673–80.

Gianoulakis, C., et al., *Different pituitary beta-endorphin and adrenal corti-sol response to ethanol in individuals with high and low risk for future development of alcoholism.* Life Sci, 1989. 45(12): pp. 1097–109.

Gianoulakis, C. and J. P. de Waele, *Genetics of alcoholism: role of the endogenous opioid system.* Metab Brain Dis, 1994. 9(2): pp. 105–31.

Gianoulakis, C., J. P. de Waele, and J. Thavundayil, *Implication of the endogenous opioid system in excessive ethanol consumption.* Alcohol, 1996. 13(1): pp. 19–23.

Giese, A. A., M. R. Thomas, and S. L. Dubovsky, *Dissociative symptoms in psychotic mood disorders: an example of symptom nonspecificty.* Psychiatry, 1997. 60(1): pp. 60–66.

Goas, J. *Endocrine factors underlying the ethanol preference of C57B1/6j mice.* Federal Proceedings, 1978 37: p. 421.

Goldfarb, A. H., and A. Z. Jamurtas, *Beta-endorphin response to exercise. An update.* Sports Med, 1997. 24(1): pp. 8–16.

Goldfarb, A. H., et al., *Gender effect on beta-endorphin response to exercise.* Med Sci Sports Exerc, 1998. 30(12): pp. 1672–6.

Gonzalez-Alonso, J., J. A. Calbet, and B. Nielsen, *Metabolic and thermo-dynamic responses to dehydration-induced reductions in muscle blood flow in exercising humans.* J Physiol, 1999. (520 Pt 2): pp. 577–89.

Grau, J. W., et al., *Long-term stress-induced analgesia and activation of the opiate system.* Science, 1981. 213(4514): pp. 1409–11.

Hainault, I., et al., *Fish oil in a high lard diet prevents obesity, hyperlipemia, and adipocyte insulin resistance in rats.* Ann NY Acad Sci, 1993. 683: pp. 98–101.

Harber, V. J., and J. R. Sutton, *Endorphins and exercise.* Sports Med, 1984. 1(2): pp. 154–71.

Harris, R. B. and H. Kor, *Insulin insensitivity is rapidly reversed in rats by reducing dietary fat from 40 to 30% of energy.* J Nutr, 1992. 122(9): pp. 1811–22.

Harte, J. L., G. H. Eifert, and R. Smith, *The effects of running and meditation on beta-endorphin, corticotropin-releasing hormone and cortisol in plasma, and on mood.* Biol Psychol, 1995. 40(3): pp. 251–65.

Hermans, B., et al., *Interaction of peptides and morphine-like narcotic analgesics with specifically labelled mu- and delta-opiate receptor binding sites.* Arch Int Pharmacodyn Ther, 1983. 263(2): pp. 317–19.

Higgins, J. A., J. C. Brand Miller, and G. S. Denyer, *Development of insulin resistance in the rat is dependent on the rate of glucose absorption from the diet.* J Nutr, 1996. 126(3): pp. 596–602.

Hill, J. O., et al., *Lipid accumulation and body fat distribution is influenced by type of dietary fat fed to rats.* Int J Obes Relat Metab Disord, 1993. 17(4): pp. 223–36.

Huang, Y. J., et al., *Amelioration of insulin resistance and hypertension in a fructose-fed rat model with fish oil supplementation.* Metabolism, 1997. 46(11): pp. 1252–8.

Jamensky, N. T., and C. Gianoulakis, *Content of dynorphins and kappa-opioid receptors in distinct brain regions of C57BL/6 and DBA/2 mice.* Alcohol Clin Exp Res, 1997. 21(8): pp. 1455–64.

Jamensky, N. T., and C. Gianoulakis, *Comparison of the proopiomelanocortin and proenkephalin opioid peptide systems in brain regions of the alcohol-preferring C57BL/6 and alcohol- avoiding DBA/2 mice.* Alcohol, 1999. 18(2–3): pp. 177–87.

Jenkins, D. D., and A. L. Jenkins, *Glycemic index and diabetes: sucrose, traditional diets and clinical utility.* J Am Coll Nutr, 1994. 13(6): pp. 541–43.

Jenkins, D. J., et al., *Glycemic index of foods: a physiological basis for carbohydrate exchange.* Am J Clin Nutr, 1981. 34(3): pp. 362–66.

Kampov-Polevoy, A., J. C. Garbutt, and D. Janowsky, *Evidence of preference for a high-concentration sucrose solution in alcoholic men.* Am J Psychiatry, 1997. 154(2): pp. 269–70.

Kampov-Polevoy, A. B., et al., *Pain sensitivity and saccharin intake in alcohol-preferring and -nonpreferring rat strains.* Physiol Behav, 1996. 59(4–5): pp. 683–88.

Kanarek, R. B., et al., *Sucrose-induced obesity: effect of diet on obesity and brown adipose tissue.* Am J Physiol, 1987. 253(1 Pt 2): pp. R158–66.

Kanarek, R. B., and N. Orthen-Gambill, *Differential effects of sucrose, fructose and glucose on carbohydrate-induced obesity in rats.* J Nutr, 1982. 112(8): pp. 1546–54.

Keith, D. E., et al., *mu-Opioid receptor internalization: opiate drugs have differential effects on a conserved endocytic mechanism in vitro and in the mammalian brain.* Mol Pharmacol, 1998. 53(3): pp. 377–84.

Kirwan, J. P., D. O'Gorman, and W. J. Evans, *A moderate glycemic meal before endurance exercise can enhance performance.* J Appl Physiol, 1998. 84(1): pp. 53–59.

Klyde, B. J., and J. Hirsch, *Increased cellular proliferation in adipose tissue of adult rats fed a high-fat diet.* J Lipid Res, 1979. 20(6): pp. 705–15.

Kolb, E., *[Recent findings in biochemistry and the significance of endorphins and enkephalins].* Z Gesamte Inn Med, 1982. 37(23): pp. 785–92.

Kraemer, R. R., et al., *Effects of treadmill running on plasma beta-endorphin, corticotropin, and cortisol levels in male and female 10K runners.* Eur J Appl Physiol Occup Phsiol, 1989. 58(8): pp. 845–51.

Kraemer, W. J., et al., *Effects of different heavy-resistance exercise protocols on plasma beta-endorphin concentrations.* J Appl Physiol, 1993. 74(1): pp. 450–59.

Kraemer, W. J., et al., *Training responses of plasma beta-endorphin, adrenocorticotropin, and cortisol.* Med Sci Sports Exerc, 1989. 21(2): pp. 146–53.

Laeng, B., K. C. Berridge, and C. M. Butter, *Pleasantness of a sweet taste during hunger and satiety: effects of gender and "sweet tooth."* Appetite, 1993. 21(3): pp. 247–54.

Lee, S. K., et al., *Defective glucose-stimulated insulin release from perifused islets of C57BL/6J mice.* Pancreas, 1995. 11(2): pp. 206–11.

Livingston, E. G., et al., *Hyperinsulinemia in the pregnant C57BL/6J mouse.* Horm Metab Res, 1994. 26(6): pp. 307–8.

Lombardo, Y. B., et al., *Dietary fish oil normalize dyslipidemia and glucose intolerance with unchanged insulin levels in rats fed a high sucrose diet.* Biochim Biophys Acta, 1996. 1299(2): pp. 175–82.

Lowinson, P. R., and R. Millman, *Substance Abuse: A Comprehensive Textbook.* 1992, Baltimore: Williams & Wilkins.

Luo, J., et al., *Dietary (n-3) polyunsaturated fatty acids improve adipocyte insulin action and glucose metabolism in insulin-resistant rats: relation to membrane fatty acids.* J Nutr, 1996. 126(8): pp. 1951–58.

Ly, A., and A. Drewnowski, *PROP (6-n-Propylthiouracil) tasting and sensory responses to caffeine, sucrose, neohesperidin dihydrochalcone and chocolate.* Chem Senses, 2001. 26(1): pp. 41–47.

Lyons, P. M., and A. S. Truswell, *Serotonin precursor influenced by type of carbohydrate meal in healthy adults.* Am J Clin Nutr, 1988. 47(3): pp. 433–39.

Maack, C., and P. Nolan, *The Effects of Guided Imagery and Music Therapy on Reported Change in Normal Adults.* J Music Ther, 1999. 36(1): pp. 39–55.

Macdiarmid, J. I., and M. M. Hetherington, *Mood modulation by food: an exploration of affect and cravings in 'chocolate addicts'.* Br J Clin Psychol, 1995. 34(Pt 1): pp. 129–38.

Marinelli, P. W., K. Kiianmaa, and C. Gianoulakis, *Opioid propeptide mRNA content and receptor density in the brains of AA and ANA rats.* Life Sci, 2000. 66(20): pp. 1915–27.

Martin, B. J., P. R. Bender, and H. Chen, *Stress hormonal response to exercise after sleep loss.* Eur J Appl Physiol Occup Physiol, 1986. 55(2): pp. 210–14.

McCubbin, J. A., et al., *Naltrexone potentiates glycemic responses during stress and epinephrine challenge in genetically obese mice.* Psychosom Med, 1989. 51(4): pp. 441–48.

McGuire, W. J., and C. V. McGuire, *Enhancing self-esteem by directed-thinking tasks: cognitive and affective positivity asymmetries.* J Pers Soc Psychol, 1996. 70(6): pp. 1117–25.

McKinney, C. H., et al., *Effects of guided imagery and music (GIM) therapy on mood and cortisol in healthy adults.* Health Psychol, 1997. 16(4): pp. 390–400.

McKinney, C. H., et al., *The effect of selected classical music and spontaneous imagery on plasma beta-endorphin.* J Behav Med, 1997. 20(1): pp. 85–99.

Mehlman, P. T., et al., *Low CSF 5-HIAA concentrations and severe aggression and impaired impulse control in nonhuman primates.* Am J Psychiatry, 1994. 151(10): pp. 1485–91.

Melchior, J. C., et al., *Immunoreactive beta-endorphin increases after an aspartame chocolate drink in healthy human subjects.* Physiol Behav, 1991. 50(5): pp. 941–4.

Morgan, W. P., *Affective beneficence of vigorous physical activity.* Med Sci Sports Exerc, 1985. 17(1): pp. 94–100.

Moskowitz, A. S., G. W. Terman, and J. C. Liebeskind, *Stress-induced analgesia in the mouse: strain comparisons.* Pain, 1985. 23(1): pp. 67–72.

Oi, Y., et al., *Allyl-containing sulfides in garlic increase uncoupling protein content in brown adipose tissue, and noradrenaline and adrenaline secretion in rats.* J Nutr, 1999. 129(2): pp. 336–42.

Okuno, M., et al., *Perilla oil prevents the excessive growth of visceral adipose tissue in rats by down-regulating adipocyte differentiation.* J Nutr, 1997. 127(9): pp. 1752–7.

Oudart, H., et al., *Brown fat thermogenesis in rats fed high-fat diets enriched with n-3 polyunsaturated fatty acids.* Int J Obes Relat Metab Disord, 1997. 21(11): pp. 955–62.

Pagliassotti, M. J., et al., *Changes in insulin action, triglycerides, and ipid composition during sucrose feeding in rats.* Am J Physiol, 1996. 271(5 Pt 2): pp. R1319–26.

Palmer, L. K., *Effects of a walking program on attributional style, depression, and self-esteem in women.* Percept Mot Skills, 1995. 81(3 Pt 1): pp. 891–98.

Panksepp, J., R. Meeker, and N. J. Bean, *The neurochemical control of crying.* Pharmacol Biochem Behav, 1980. 12(3): pp. 437–43.

Parekh, P. I., et al., *Reversal of diet-induced obesity and diabetes in C57BL/6J mice.* Metabolism, 1998. 47(9): pp. 1089–96.

Parrish, C. C., D. A. Pathy, and A. Angel, *Dietary fish oils limit adipose tissue hypertrophy in rats.* Metabolism, 1990. 39(3): pp. 217–9.

Parrish, C. C., et al., *Dietary fish oils modify adipocyte structure and function.* J Cell Physiol, 1991. 148(3): pp. 493–502.

Pavlicevic, M., and C. Trevarthen, *A musical assessment of psychiatric states in adults.* Psychopathology, 1989. 22(6): pp. 325–34.

Pennington, J., *Food Values of Portions Commonly Used.* 1994, Philadelphia: J.B. Lippincott Co.

Pert, A., R. Simantov, and S. H. Snyder, *A morphine-like factor in mammalian brain: analgesic activity in rats.* Brain Res, 1977. 136(3): pp. 523–33.

Pert, C. B., A. Pert, and J. F. Tallman, *Isolation of a novel endogenous opiate analgesic from human blood.* Proc Natl Acad Sci U S A, 1976. 73(7): pp. 2226–30.

Petty, F., G. Kramer, and M. Moeller, *Does learned helplessness induction by haloperidol involve serotonin mediation?* Pharmacol Biochem Behav, 1994. 48(3): pp. 671–76.

Petty, F., G. L. Kramer, and J. Wu, *Serotonergic modulation of learned helplessness.* Ann NY Acad Sci, 1997. 821: pp. 538–41.

Petty, F., et al., *Posttraumatic stress and depression. A neurochemical anatomy of the learned helplessness animal model.* Ann N Y Acad Sci, 1997. 821: pp. 529–32.

Pierce, E. F., et al., *Resistance exercise decreases beta-endorphin immunoreactivity.* Br J Sports Med, 1994. 28(3): pp. 164–66.

Pierce, E. F., et al., *Beta-endorphin response to endurance exercise: relationship to exercise dependence.* Percept Mot Skills, 1993. 77(3 Pt 1): pp. 767–70.

Ponnampalam, E. N., et al., *Effect of dietary modification of muscle long-chain n-3 fatty acid on plasma insulin and lipid metabolites, carcass traits, and fat deposition in lambs.* J Anim Sci, 2001. 79(4): pp. 895–903.

Prerost, F. J., *Reduction of aggression as a function of related content of humor.* Psychol Rep, 1976. 38(3 pt. 1): pp. 771–77.

Prerost, F. J., *Presentation of humor and facilitation of a relaxation response among internal and external scorers on Rotter's scale.* Psychol Rep, 1993. 72(3 Pt 2): pp. 1248–50.

Prerost, F. J., *Humor preferences among angered males and females: associations with humor content and sexual desire.* Psychol Rep, 1995. 77(1): pp. 227–34.

Przewlocka, B., et al., *The difference in stress-induced analgesia in C57BL/6 and DBA/2 mice: a search for biochemical correlates.* Pol J Pharmacol Pharm, 1988. 40(5): pp. 497–506.

Rahkila, P., et al., *Beta-endorphin and corticotropin release is dependent on a threshold intensity of running exercise in male endurance athletes.* Life Sci, 1988. 43(6): pp. 551–58.

Rahkila, P., et al., *Response of plasma endorphins to running exercises in male and female endurance athletes.* Med Sci Sports Exerc, 1987. 19(5): pp. 451–55.

Reaven, G. M., *Role of insulin resistance in human disease (syndrome X): an expanded definition.* Annu Rev Med, 1993. 44: pp. 121–31.

Reaven, G. M., *Insulin resistance and human disease: a short history.* J Basic Clin Physiol Pharmacol, 1998. 9(2–4): pp. 387–406.

Rider, M. S., J. W. Floyd, and J. Kirkpatrick, *The effect of music, therapy, and relaxation on adrenal corticosteroids and the re-entrainment of circadian rhythms.* J Music Ther, 1985. 22(1): pp. 46–58.

Roy, A., M. Virkkunen, and M. Linnoila, *Monoamines, glucose metabolism, aggression towards self and others.* Int J Neurosci, 1988. 41(3–4): pp. 261–64.

Sakamoto, H., et al.,[*Individual differences in image and pulse-wave responses elicited by listening to music*]. Nippon Eiseigaku Zasshi, 1991. 45(6): pp. 1053–60.

Schwarz, L., and W. Kindermann, *Changes in beta-endorphin levels in response to aerobic and anaerobic exercise.* Sports Med, 1992. 13(1): pp. 25–36.

Sforzo, G. A., *Opioids and exercise.* An update. Sports Med, 1989. 7(2): pp. 109–24.

Shalev, A. Y., T. Galai, and S. Eth, *Levels of trauma: a multidimensional approach to the treatment of PTSD.* Psychiatry, 1993. 56(2): pp. 166–77.

Sherman, W. M., M. C. Peden, and D. A. Wright, *Carbohydrate feedings 1 h before exercise improves cycling performance.* Am J Clin Nutr, 1991. 54(5): pp. 866–70.

Shimomura, Y., T. Tamura, and M. Suzuki, *Less body fat accumulation in rats fed a safflower oil diet than in rats fed a beef tallow diet.* J Nutr, 1990. 120(11): pp. 1291–6.

Simoneau, J. A., J. H. Veerkamp, L. P. Turcotte, and D. E. Kelley, *Markers of capacity to utilize fatty acids in human skeletal muscle: relation to insulin resistance and obesity and effects of weight loss.* FASEB J, 1999. 13(14): pp. 2051–60.

Snyder, S. H., *The opiate receptor and morphine-like peptides in the brain.* Am J Psychiatry, 1978. 135(6): pp. 645–52.

Southgate, D. A., *Digestion and metabolism of sugars.* Am J Clin Nutr, 1995. 62(1 Suppl): pp. 203S–210S; discussion 211S.

Stewart, R., *Consumption of sweet, salty, sour, and bitter solutions by selectively bred alcohol-preferring and alcohol-nonpreferring lines of rats.* Alcoholism: Clinical and Experimental Research, 1994. 18(2): pp. 375–81.

Storlien, L. H., et al., *Fish oil prevents insulin resistance induced by high-fat feeding in rats.* Science, 1987. 237(4817): pp. 885–88.

Sumova, A. and B. Jakoubek, *Analgesia and impact induced by anticipation stress: involvement of the endogenous opioid peptide system.* Brain Res, 1989. 503(2): pp. 273–80.

Surwit, R. S., and S. Collins, *Revisiting lessons from the C57BL/6J mouse.* Am J Physiol Endocrinol Metab, 2001. 280(5): pp. E825–26.

Surwit, R. S., et al., *Transient effects of long-term leptin supplementation in the prevention of diet-induced obesity in mice.* Diabetes, 2000. 49(7): pp. 1203–8.

Surwit, R. S., and M. N. Feinglos, *The effects of relaxations on glucose tolerance in non-insulin-dependent diabetes.* Diabetes Care, 1983. 6(2): pp. 176–9.

Surwit, R. S., et al., *Metabolic and behavioral effects of a high-sucrose diet during weight loss.* Am J Clin Nutr, 1997. 65(4): pp. 908–15.

Surwit, R. S., et al., *Differential effects of fat and sucrose on the development of obesity and diabetes in C57BL/6J and A/J mice.* Metabolism, 1995. 44(5): pp. 645–51.

Surwit, R. S., et al., *Diet-induced type II diabetes in C57BL/6J mice.* Diabetes, 1988. 37(9): pp. 1163–7.

Surwit, R. S., et al., *Differential glycemic effects of morphine in diabetic and normal mice.* Metabolism, 1989. 38(3): pp. 282–85.

Surwit, R. S., et al., *Low plasma leptin in response to dietary fat in diabetes- and obesity-prone mice.* Diabetes, 1997. 46(9): pp. 1516–20.

Surwit, R. S., et al., *Control of expression of insulin resistance and hyperglycemia by different genetic factors in diabetic C57BL/6J mice.* Diabetes, 1991. 40(1): pp. 82–87.

Surwit, R. S., et al., *Diet-induced changes in uncoupling proteins in obesity-prone and obesity-resistant strains of mice.* Proc Natl Acad Sci USA, 1998. 95(7): pp. 4061–5.

Takeuchi, H., et al., *Diet-induced thermogenesis is lower in rats fed a lard diet than in those fed a high oleic acid safflower oil diet, a safflower oil diet or a linseed oil diet.* J Nutr, 1995. 125(4): pp. 920–25.

Tejedor-Real, P., et al., *Implication of endogenous opioid system in the learned helplessness model of depression.* Pharmacol Biochem Behav, 1995. 52(1): pp. 145–52.

Tejedor-Real, P., et al., *Involvement of delta-opioid receptors in the effects induced by endogenous enkephalins on learned helplessness model.* Eur J Pharmacol, 1998. 354(1): pp. 1–7.

Terjung, R. L., *Muscle fiber involvement during training of different intensities and durations.* Am J Physiol, 1976. 230(4): pp. 946–50.

Thompson, M. L., et al., *Analgesia in defeated mice: evidence for mediation via central rather than pituitary or adrenal endogenous opioid peptides.* Pharmacol Biochem Behav, 1988. 29(3): pp. 451–56.

van der Kolk, B. A., *The body keeps the score: memory and the evolving psychobiology of posttraumatic stress.* Harv Rev Psychiatry, 1994. 1(5): pp. 253–65.

van der Kolk, B. A., et al., *Endogenous opioids, stress induced analgesia, and posttraumatic stress disorder.* Psychopharmacol Bull, 1989. 25(3): pp. 417–21.

van der Kolk, B. A., et al., *Trauma and the development of borderline personality disorder.* Psychiatr Clin North Am, 1994. 17(4): pp. 715–30.

Virkkunen, M., *Reactive hypoglycemic tendency among habitually violent offenders.* Nutr Rev, 1986. 44 Suppl: pp. 94–103.

Virkkunen, M., et al., *Cerebrospinal fluid monoamine metabolite levels in male arsonists.* Arch Gen Psychiatry, 1987. 44(3): pp. 241–47.

Wencel, H. E., et al., *Impaired second phase insulin response of diabetes-prone C57BL/6J mouse islets.* Physiol Behav, 1995. 57(6): pp. 1215–20.

Wildmann, J., et al., *Increase of circulating beta-endorphin-like immunoreactivity correlates with the change in feeling of pleasantness after running.* Life Sci, 1986. 38(11): pp. 997–1003.

Will, M. J., L. R. Watkins, and S. F. Maier, *Uncontrollable stress potentiates morphine's rewarding properties.* Pharmacol Biochem Behav, 1998. 60(3): pp. 655–64.

Wolever, T. M., et al., *The glycemic index: methodology and clinical implications.* Am J Clin Nutr, 1991. 54(5): pp. 846–54.

Wolever, T. M., et al., *Beneficial effect of low-glycemic index diet in overweight NIDDM subjects.* Diabetes Care, 1992. 15(4): pp. 562–64.

Wu, J., et al., *Serotonin and learned helplessness: a regional study of 5-HT1A, 5-HT2A receptors and the serotonin transport site in rat brain.* J Psychiatr Res, 1999. 33(1): pp. 17–22.

Wurtman, J. J., *Carbohydrate craving. Relationship between carbohydrate intake and disorders of mood.* Drugs, 1990. 39(Suppl 3): pp. 49–52.

Wurtman, R. J., and J. J. Wurtman, *Brain serotonin, carbohydrate-craving, obesity and depression.* Obes Res, 1995. 3 Suppl 4: pp. 477S–480S.

Ziegler, P. J., et al., *Body image and dieting behaviors among elite figure skaters.* Int J Eat Disord, 1998. 24(4): pp. 421–27.

Zorrilla, E. P., R. J. DeRubeis, and E. Redei, *High self-esteem, hardiness and affective stability are associated with higher basal pituitary-adrenal hormone levels.* Psychoneuroendocrinology, 1995. 20(6): pp. 591–601.

Index

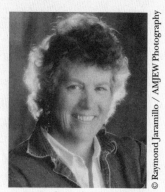

About the Author

KATHLEEN DESMAISONS, Ph.D., coined the term "sugar sensitivity" to describe a unique biochemical profile that appears to be a gate to addiction and compulsive behavior. Dr. DesMaisons started the field of Addictive Nutrition in 1996 and is now recognized as the leading expert in the use of nutrition to heal the biochemistry of addiction. Dr. DesMaisons is the president and CEO of Radiant Recovery, an international online treatment program for alcoholism, addiction, depression, and other self-destructive compulsive behaviors. Her website www.radiantrecovery.com serves hundreds of thousands and has had more than 10 million hits. It provides more than sixty special support lists for sugar-sensitive people recovering from alcoholism and bulimia, and covering topics such as fitness, chronic illness, book study, journaling, parents, children, teens, friends and families, and even the pets of participants.

Dr. DesMaisons has authored *Potatoes Not Prozac* and *The Sugar Addict's Total Recovery Program*.

Dr. DesMaisons resides in Albuquerque, New Mexico.

For More Information

If you would like to learn more about healing sugar sensitivity and opportunities for weight loss

Call toll free: (888) 579-3970
Online: www.radiantrecovery.com
Email: admin@radiantrecovery.com

You can order George's Shake® or audio tapes of any of Dr. DesMaisons' books online or by the toll free number.